T0260919

Training to Change Practice

Training to Change Practice

Behavioural Science to Develop Effective Health Professional Education

Jo Hart

Professor of Health Professional Education
University of Manchester, UK

Lucie Byrne-Davis

Professor of Health Psychology
University of Manchester, UK

Wendy Maltinsky

Health Psychology Senior Lecturer
University of Stirling, UK

Eleanor Bull

Senior Health Psychologist, Manchester University
NHS Foundation Trust, UK

Highly Specialised Health Psychologist, Derbyshire
County Council, UK

Honorary Senior Lecturer, University of Manchester, UK

WILEY Blackwell

This edition first published 2023
© 2023 John Wiley & Sons Ltd

All rights reserved. No part of this publication may be reproduced, stored in a retrieval system, or transmitted, in any form or by any means, electronic, mechanical, photocopying, recording or otherwise, except as permitted by law. Advice on how to obtain permission to reuse material from this title is available at http://www.wiley.com/go/permissions.

The right of Jo Hart, Lucie Byrne-Davis, Wendy Maltinsky and Eleanor Bull to be identified as the authors of this work / the editorial material in this work has been asserted in accordance with law.

Registered Office(s)
John Wiley & Sons, Inc., 111 River Street, Hoboken, NJ 07030, USA
John Wiley & Sons Ltd, The Atrium, Southern Gate, Chichester, West Sussex, PO19 8SQ, UK

Editorial Office
9600 Garsington Road, Oxford, OX4 2DQ, UK

For details of our global editorial offices, customer services, and more information about Wiley products visit us at www.wiley.com.

Wiley also publishes its books in a variety of electronic formats and by print-on-demand. Some content that appears in standard print versions of this book may not be available in other formats.

Limit of Liability/Disclaimer of Warranty
The contents of this work are intended to further general scientific research, understanding, and discussion only and are not intended and should not be relied upon as recommending or promoting scientific method, diagnosis, or treatment by physicians for any particular patient. In view of ongoing research, equipment modifications, changes in governmental regulations, and the constant flow of information relating to the use of medicines, equipment, and devices, the reader is urged to review and evaluate the information provided in the package insert or instructions for each medicine, equipment, or device for, among other things, any changes in the instructions or indication of usage and for added warnings and precautions. While the publisher and authors have used their best efforts in preparing this work, they make no representations or warranties with respect to the accuracy or completeness of the contents of this work and specifically disclaim all warranties, including without limitation any implied warranties of merchantability or fitness for a particular purpose. No warranty may be created or extended by sales representatives, written sales materials or promotional statements for this work. The fact that an organization, website, or product is referred to in this work as a citation and/or potential source of further information does not mean that the publisher and authors endorse the information or services the organization, website, or product may provide or recommendations it may make. This work is sold with the understanding that the publisher is not engaged in rendering professional services. The advice and strategies contained herein may not be suitable for your situation. You should consult with a specialist where appropriate. Further, readers should be aware that websites listed in this work may have changed or disappeared between when this work was written and when it is read. Neither the publisher nor authors shall be liable for any loss of profit or any other commercial damages, including but not limited to special, incidental, consequential, or other damages.

A catalogue record for this book is available from the Library of Congress

Paperback ISBN: 9781119833482; ePub ISBN: 9781394172214; ePDF ISBN: 9781119833499; oBook ISBN: 9781119833505

Cover Image: © beanimages/Shutterstock
Cover Design: Wiley

Set in 10.5/13 pt STIXTwoText by Integra Software Services Pvt. Ltd, Pondicherry, India
Printed and bound by CPI Group (UK) Ltd, Croydon, CR0 4YY

C9781119833482_300123

Contents

Foreword

This first edition of *Training to Change Practice* is a jewel for educators, psychologists and scientists. The four co-authors – the JEWeL of Jo, Eleanor, Wendy and Lucie – have drawn upon their domestic and international experiences to identify and propose practical solutions to one of the most salient issues in health and care systems worldwide: the market failures in the conceptualization, development, delivery and impact of education and training for health and care workers.

The authors rightly open chapter 1, and inform the book throughout, with an appreciation of health professional's education and training as an economic sector, an industry, a market: with its inherent strengths and weaknesses and highly susceptible to internal and external factors. Their evidence from Canada and the United Kingdom strongly resonates with reviews and commissioned studies from the World Health Organization that conservatively estimate global expenditure in lifelong learning in the health and care economy in the range of US$12-15 billion per annum. A market that – when subject to scrutiny, evaluation and scientific review – demonstrates limited effect on practice and patient outcomes, irrespective of whether training is delivered in low-, middle- or high-income settings.

This global market within health and care systems has grown decade by decade: heavily influenced by two factors. A belief among many that "in-service training" was the primary solution to address quality of health services through improving the skills and knowledge of the health and care workforce, and secondly the expansion of official development assistance to health in the period from 2000.

Fortunately, the increased spending on in-service training has also generated additional analysis and scrutiny. In particular, multi-disciplinary teams of behavioural, education and health systems' specialists are increasingly combining their respective sciences to reveal the conceptual flaws in the theory of change and bring new thinking to the fore. This contemporary logic includes moving beyond the transfer of knowledge, the assessment of time allocated to study, or the measurement of learners' satisfaction with the training experience to one of how adults learn, their behaviour in teams and institutions, and how to develop competencies that will be routinely applied in practice. Assessment and learning transfer evaluation models likewise focus on the demonstrable application of learning.

Similar concepts are very much evident in this book, where the authors' collective wisdom – channelled convincingly through "we believe", "we find", "we argue" and "we propose" statements – focuses on practical techniques, measures and theories of behavioural science to impact change in the workplace.

The book opens with a short overview of applicable concepts and theories, and the simple COM-B framework (*capability, opportunity, motivation -> behaviour*) that underpins subsequent chapters, before introducing seven key principles to develop and inform effective training. Chapters 2, 3 and 4 then guide the reader through a step-by-step approach to how to apply behavioural science techniques before Chapter 5 sets out a pragmatic approach to assessing and evaluating change, drawing upon process and outcome measurement. Many readers will particularly enjoy the topic guides, tips and examples and sample training plans across the book.

Beyond presenting the complexity of the field in an informative and instructional format, the co-authors challenge and nudge the reader to learn, think and act differently in their practice. Whilst drawing upon a rich, collective experience of the United Kingdom's National Health Service with some examples from less resourced settings it is a public good for international application.

The book is particularly timely given the global health challenges arising from three years of the COVID19 pandemic. Many health and care systems are facing reductions in government health expenditure in real terms, new demands to recover, 'build back better' and expand preparedness in health security, and increasing political and financial pressure on health providers to optimize existing resources in pursuit of effective, quality services. Inevitably these demands will be transferred to the millions of health and care teams around the world to solve; requiring concerted efforts to invest in competency-based, behaviourally informed training that targets changes in practice.

All parties involved in the commissioning, subsidy, development and delivery of lifelong learning targeted to health and care professionals' can learn much from this book. The application of the principles, tools and approach would do much to accelerate the use of behavioural science in the training of the world's health and care workforce, address existing market failures and impact learning, practice and patient outcomes.

Jim Campbell
Director, Health Workforce
World Health Organization

Acknowledgements

We would like to thank Association for the Study of Medical Education for their support in the development of this book. Also, we would like to thank all the wonderful clinical educators we have worked with and particularly our colleagues at Health Education England, Tropical Health & Education Trust and Advanced Life Support Group.

We are very grateful to our supportive health psychology community, in particular The Change Exchange, Chris Armitage, Justin Presseau, Nicola McCleary, Jeremy Grimshaw and Marie Johnston.

With thanks to Paul Davis for expert proof reading.

CHAPTER 1

Education and Training as a Behaviour Change Intervention

Jo Hart[1], Lucie Byrne-Davis[2], Wendy Maltinsky[3], Eleanor Bull[4,5,6], Nicola McCleary[7] and Chris Armitage[8]

[1] Professor of Health Professional Education, University of Manchester, UK
[2] Professor of Health Psychology, University of Manchester, UK
[3] Health Psychology Senior Lecturer, University of Stirling, UK
[4] Senior Health Psychologist, Manchester University NHS Foundation Trust, UK
[5] Highly Specialised Health Psychologist, Derbyshire County Council, UK
[6] Honorary Senior Lecturer, University of Manchester, UK
[7] Senior Implementation Research Fellow, Ottawa Hospital Research Institute, Canada
[8] Professor of Health Psychology, University of Manchester, UK

Learning Points

- Education and training can be an intervention to change healthcare practice
- Clinical practice is composed of multiple behaviours, such as diagnosis, treatment and management, monitoring and supporting self-management

Training to Change Practice: Behavioural Science to Develop Effective Health Professional Education, First Edition. Jo Hart, Lucie Byrne-Davis, Wendy Maltinsky, and Eleanor Bull.
© 2023 John Wiley & Sons Ltd. Published 2023 by John Wiley & Sons Ltd.

- Practice behaviours are influenced by capability, opportunity and motivation
- There are theory- and evidence-based methods to increase the likelihood of clinical practice change

WHAT IS CONTINUING PROFESSIONAL DEVELOPMENT?

Continuing professional development (CPD) is an umbrella term, covering all kinds of activities that help health professionals learn and develop throughout their careers (e.g., Peck et al. 2000). Among the most widespread CPD activities are the structured education opportunities that we will describe in this book as CPD training courses, although they are also called educational meetings or workshops (Forsetlund et al. 2021). As long ago as 2002, the UK NHS was estimated to directly spend approximately £1 billion annually on workforce CPD (Brown et al. 2002). CPD is seen as crucial to developing the more flexible, multidisciplinary health workforce envisioned in the recent NHS Long Term Plan (Karas et al. 2020). Given how much is invested in CPD, it is even more important that CPD is designed to maximise practice improvement, so the benefits of investment can be fully realised in terms of improving care delivery and ultimately health outcomes.

THE PURPOSE(S) OF CPD

In healthcare (and social care) settings, the main aim of CPD is to maintain and improve standards of safe and effective care. For instance, the Health and Care Professions Council, one of the nine regulators of the UK health professional workforce, define CPD to ensure practitioners 'keep their skills and knowledge up to date and are able to practise safely and effectively' (HCPC 2022). CPD may also aim to increase staff motivation, well-being and retention (Brown et al. 2002) through supporting staff to form new networks, feel valued, meet their personal development needs and benefit from reflective time away from their usual roles. This all sounds fantastic in theory, but as educators ourselves working to organise a wide range of CPD in the UK and internationally, we have found that developing training that changes hearts and minds, and most importantly, practice, is not all that easy. Research agrees: a recent Cochrane review combining 215 studies of educational meetings for healthcare professionals found these to only slightly improve professional practice compared to no intervention, with even fewer effects on patient outcomes (Forsetlund et al. 2021). Indeed, despite the aim of CPD being to improve and maintain safe and effective care, a review of accredited CPD activities offered to health professionals in

Canada showed that 96% of the learning objectives targeted changes in cognition, i.e. were not designed to promote practice change (Légaré et al. 2015).

THE CHALLENGES OF CHANGING PRACTICE THROUGH CPD

If you have ever led a CPD training, you may have some examples of challenges you have come across. We describe some examples below from our own experience. Through talking to others, we think these types of challenges are quite common. Imagine that you have just wrapped up a one-day training course, teaching hospital staff to use structured assessment approaches to handle medical emergencies. You're packing away the handouts, feeling pretty happy with all the positive feedback forms. Staff members come up to you and tell you that 'It was amazing! We loved it! Thank you and please come back again for more!' but that 'of course, we can't do any of those things in *our* clinic...'. What about training a group of community health improvement workers to use a new communication tool with families? They're nodding and smiling in all the right places; it seems to be going well, but then you mention the fateful words 'role play', their arms fold and they frowningly say 'oh no, in our team, we don't *do* role play...'. What if a colleague tells you they don't think CPD should aim to change practice, that this is 'paternalistic' and practitioners should not be 'manipulated into changing what they do'?

Maybe you've worked hard for the last few months doing hand hygiene training across your hospital and you're thrilled that you've trained so many people. Then the audit figures come in and frustration of frustrations... staff hand hygiene compliance is the same as it was before! You can feel like all your efforts have been like stirring water in a bucket – you can see the water swirling and rippling at the time, but as soon as you stop, the water settles and it's like your hand was never there.

As psychologists working in multidisciplinary teams (MDT) with colleagues from different professional backgrounds, we and our MDT colleagues believe that behavioural science might hold some of the answers to challenging training situations. In this book, we offer a guide to developing engaging training which is grounded in a deep understanding of learners' practice and its drivers, uses behavioural science theory and evidence-based tailored training techniques and takes a behavioural approach to evaluation.

In this chapter, we will introduce you to some of the robust theory and methods underpinning this approach, particularly the Behaviour Change Wheel method (Michie, van Stralen and West 2011) developed in the past decade. Following this, in Chapter 2, we will focus on how to identify and specify the multiple behaviours that your training aims to change. Chapter

3 will introduce methods to help you understand what helps and gets in the way of helping health professionals to carry out these behaviours. These behavioural influences will be targets for your training. We will explore, in Chapter 4, a step-by-step approach to using the information about behaviours and their influences to develop targeted, engaging training approaches. Finally, in Chapter 5, we will explore how to assess learners' progress and evaluate training meaningfully using behavioural science methods. We hope that this book, built on a good foundation of educational principles and folding in some behavioural science, will help you to create CPD that is ready to fly, just like our cover image.

Many of these ideas are as old as the behavioural theories underpinning them (up to 150 years). We hope that educators will recognise much good practice that they already do, as well as offering a space to reflect on times like those examples above where things didn't go so well. The book aims to offer opportunities to mindfully experiment with change in your CPD, from small tweaks to creating behaviourally informed CPD from the outset. We welcome readers to get in touch with thoughts and experiences as they try out ideas. Working closely with our MDT colleagues and at the research-practice boundary is how we all will keep building the science on how to develop training which offers learners a positive experience, builds confidence, motivation, knowledge and skills, and most importantly enables learners to translate this into improvements in their practice back in their real-life work setting.

IMPORTANT CONCEPTS AND THEORIES

Miller's Pyramid

Miller's Pyramid is famous in medical education (Miller 1990). Figure 1 neatly shows the building blocks of performance from 'knowing', 'knowing how', through 'showing how' and all the way to 'does'. Miller's model has been hugely influential, shaping educational curricula and approaches to assessment of professional competencies in spheres far beyond medicine (Cruess et al. 2016).

Undoubtedly, in order to do something, someone must almost always know how to do it (the exception being things that we do of which we are not aware). Does it follow, though, that if someone knows how to do something and *can* actually do it (show how) that they *will* do it in practice? Behavioural science tells us that just because someone *can* do something does not

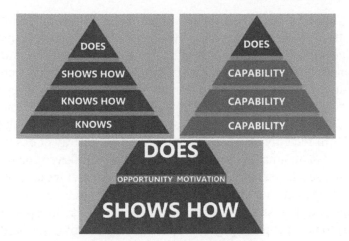

FIGURE 1   The interaction of capability, opportunity, motivation and Miller's Pyramid. The first diagram (top left) shows Miller's Pyramid, the second (top right) that most of Miller's (knows, knows how, shows how) is capability, the third (bottom) that opportunity and motivation can move us between 'shows how' and 'does'.

mean that they **will**. So, how does behavioural science fit with Miller's Pyramid? Firstly, there are techniques in behavioural science that can be used to move people from 'can do' to 'does'. There are many of them, and we will cover some of them in Chapter 4, when we discuss developing training to change practice. These sorts of techniques are sometimes present in education and training but are less often and less explicitly used than techniques to develop knowledge and skills (Pearson et al. 2020). Secondly, educators typically evaluate the efficacy of their training through measures of knowledge and skill, meaning that there is much less focus in quality assurance, quality improvement and educational evaluation, on how 'shows how' becomes 'does', i.e. does the education go beyond changing what you **can** do to what you **actually** do.

Educators do, of course, focus on changing more than knowledge and skills in their teaching. Many CPD activities will begin with a clinical case illustrating the need for change and perhaps research evidence highlighting improved outcomes with changed practice. In fact, when we studied different types of CPD, we found over 40 behaviour change techniques (Pearson et al. 2020). Some activities will involve reflection, in which trainees will be asked to think about barriers to adopting the new practices. Implicit in these activities is an underlying theory of how behaviour changes and the techniques or methods of achieving changes in professional practice.

Psychologists and other behavioural scientists have been researching for decades the all-important question: 'How and when do people translate new knowledge and skills gained in training or other interventions into action?' One problem in studying this is one of language. Imagine you were a medical scientist and had developed a new wonder drug. Using established frameworks like the periodic table you'd be able to tell people exactly what was in it (although no doubt your lips would be sealed until you had it patented!). Until recently, behavioural scientists had no way of describing the 'ingredients' of an amazing new behavioural health intervention or training course because one person might describe an activity as, for example, offering 'social support', whilst another might call it 'giving encouragement' or even 'arranging a bus to take people to the training venue!' (a more practical form of support to help people engage in training). This meant it was hard to build the evidence of 'what works, for whom' – lots of teams would try to evaluate the effectiveness of training, but were not necessarily talking about the same thing.

A SHARED THEORETICAL LANGUAGE

The benefits of having a shared language should not be underestimated. Behavioural scientists have made attempts to develop a shared language by developing a behaviour change technique taxonomy (Michie et al. 2013) that names and describes the techniques used by educators and others to change behaviour; over 90 behaviour change methods were identified. Our finding, that around 40 of these techniques were used in health professional education and training, (Pearson et al. 2020) suggests that educators are currently not exploiting their full potential.

Behavioural science has a wide range of theories which outline that both conscious (e.g., intentions, goals) and unconscious (e.g., habits) processes influence behaviour, but CPD activities aimed at changing behaviour tend to be restricted to addressing conscious, reflective thoughts and attitudes. Healthcare professional behaviour, like most human behaviour, is influenced by both types of process: not just what we believe but also our emotions, needs and habits (habit is part of automatic motivation) (Eccles et al. 2012). For example, in one study of GPs in the UK, those who had the strongest habits of giving weight advice, examining feet and prescribing blood pressure reducing drugs did this most often in their practice 12 months later (Presseau et al. 2014). This can mean prompting behaviour by what has commonly come to be known as a 'nudge' (Thaler and Sunstein 2021). In a recent review of Cochrane Reviews of 'nudge strategies' to improve health workers' implementation of guidelines, nudge strategies were found to be equivalent to other interventions targeting implementation of guidelines (Yoong et al. 2020). In other words, our automatic processes can and do influence how we practise at work and so should be considered if we want to change practice. We will think more about what we can do in education and training to influence automatic processes in Chapter 4.

WHY THINK ABOUT BEHAVIOURAL THEORY?

So, back to thinking about theory. Why are we interested in it? Good theory can have practical benefits but only if communicated effectively. Theory enhances understanding of behaviour, offers a summary of the evidence on what drives behaviour, and proposes opportunities for intervention to achieve the desired behaviours and consequent health benefits (Michie et al. 2014). However, the benefits in practice might be limited by complexity, the vast number of theories available, and a lack of shared language. An early attempt at simplification (Michie et al. 2005) increased the use of behavioural science theory in the implementation of evidence-based practice.

The behavioural science literature has remained largely untouched by the healthcare professional education communities. There are, of course, notable exceptions (Cilliers et al. 2015) but largely, in education and training, the translation of abilities into practice is seen as beyond the borders of the classroom or skills lab and, therefore, beyond the realm of the educator. On the other hand, in healthcare journals, there are numerous papers reporting attempts to change practice of healthcare professionals, for example, in the case of hand hygiene (Luangasanatip et al. 2015, McCay 2015). The shared goal of these 'complex interventions' and 'education and training' is practice change to bring about some improvement in health or care. However, one type of activity arises from 'education' whilst the other arises from 'implementation' or 'quality improvement'. We would argue that there is efficacy and efficiency benefits from bringing these two types together. In our work in multidisciplinary teams, we have found that a recent framework, The COM-B Framework, makes the main ideas of behavioural science accessible to educators and trainers.

THE COM-B FRAMEWORK

There are many theories of behaviour that use different descriptions of the same theoretical constructs. It is difficult for anyone to choose a theory and at least 83 theories of behaviour change relevant for designing interventions to change behaviour have been identified (Michie et al. 2014). In the last couple of decades, there have been some attempts to synthesise theories into overarching frameworks. In our own work, when we work directly with educators and trainers, we find using the COM-B framework (Michie et al. 2011) to be a simple and effective way of describing the multiple influences on behaviour (see Figure 2 for examples). Of course, each of C, O and M are umbrella terms for the complexity of influences but they are a good place to start.

Capability is both physical and psychological which include skills and knowledge respectively and also includes decision making about enacting behaviours, choosing between alternatives, cognitive abilities in retaining and applying specific information, and abilities to focus; as well as capabilities to self-monitor behaviour and self-enact change strategies.

'*I know it*', '*I know how to do it*' and '*I can show how to do it*' (see Figure 1).

Opportunity is both physical and social. Physical opportunity covers things in your environment like having time, funding and the right equipment. Social opportunity is best summarised as 'the way we do things round here' and is sometimes known as 'culture', 'peer pressure' or 'hidden curriculum'.

'*I have everything I need to do it*' and '*people whose opinion I care about think I should do it*'.

Motivation is both reflective and automatic. Reflective motivation is when people weigh up the pros and cons of the behaviour and will include

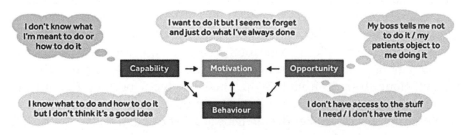

FIGURE 2   Influences on behaviour mapped to capability, opportunity and motivation.

things like whether they think the behaviour will lead to a good end point, whether the behaviour is difficult or easy or whether they feel in control of doing the behaviour. Automatic motivation includes impulses to carry out the behaviour, our emotions and drives and includes things like habit and conditioning.

'On balance I think it is a good idea' and *'It is part of my usual practice'*, *'it makes me feel good'* and *'I just do it without really thinking too much about it'.*

A FOCUS ON MOTIVATION

Motivation is a complex construct. Within the COM-B Framework, motivation is both reflective and automatic. Behavioural scientists will talk about 'dual process theories' which explain how reflective and automatic motivation interact to influence behaviour (Evans 2008). In health, the system 1 (automatic) – system 2 (reflective) dual process theory (Kahneman 2011) is often used when discussing human factors in patient safety. For example, 'I plan to ask diabetes patients about their feet, and I place a tag on all of their notes that pops up through the consultation which acts as a reminder'. A full exploration of these theories is beyond the scope of this book but there is some further reading at the end of this chapter. PRIME Theory of Motivation is a useful way to think about how our reflective and automatic processes come together in the moment causing us to do – or not do – key behaviours (West and Brown 2014). PRIME Theory brings reflective and automatic processes into one model, discussing that our behaviours at every moment are governed by potentially competing impulses and inhibitions. These in turn arise from motives/desires and our instinctive and learned associations, i.e. what we have learnt to do in that situation and what we instinctively do in that situation. If we think about PRIME Theory then we can start to realise why people might be really motivated to do something when they think about it outside of their normal work, but then fail to do it when they are back at work. In other words, it helps us to understand why people can leave a CPD training course full of energy and intentions, and then not make any changes to what they do every day. We like this perspective because the evidence supports it, but also because it makes us all less judgemental about our own practice or that of others. Instead, it focuses our mind on how CPD can be used to support change in people who want to make that change.

WHY IS BEHAVIOURAL SCIENCE IMPORTANT?

Education and training in health professional education and CPD is often explicitly focused on improving competence. Indeed, competency-based education for health professionals is an international gold standard (World Health Organisation 2022). In Figure 1, we see how these behavioural influences of capability, opportunity and motivation can be demonstrated by looking at and re-labelling Miller's Pyramid.

Our own work coding CPD courses for behaviour change techniques found that educators most often used those focused on improving capability (Pearson et al. 2020). Whilst it is crucial to focus on competence, we propose that this leads to a lost opportunity for health professional education and training. Specifically, we propose that deliberately thinking about the opportunity and the motivation of health professionals allows educators to a) use a wider variety of techniques and b) evaluate changes in the whole set of factors that drive behaviour. Further, it supports educators accessing and learning from research that is called something different (like implementation or improvement or complex interventions) but is attempting to achieve the same outcomes.

In the following chapters, we present a series of practical suggestions for how education and training can incorporate techniques, measures and theories of behavioural science, starting with developing a comprehensive theory of change. Before we do that, we wanted to mention other important psychological aspects of education and training.

EFFECTIVE AND ENJOYABLE TRAINING

In this book, we will talk about some of the 'active ingredients' of interventions to change practice that have been studied by behavioural scientists in many settings, such as goal setting. However, we all know from our own experience that someone can help us set goals in a helpful, encouraging way, drawing out what is important to us and inspiring and motivating us to reach for them... or in much less helpful ways. In this way, a training course is much more than the 'sum of its parts'. We need to bring our more holistic understanding of how human psychology and how people learn to the fore. These come out in the key principles for effective training below.

PRINCIPLES FOR EFFECTIVE TRAINING

We apply several key principles in our educational activities, grounded in pedagogical and behavioural science.

Principle 1. Starting from Where Learners Are

In many educational courses, the myth of 'learning styles' still prevails, the idea that it is useful to align instruction to learners' particular preferred 'style' of delivery (e.g., listening, seeing or physically doing activities). Psychological and pedagogical research has consistently shown that there is no benefit in tailoring teaching to so-called learning styles (Kirschner 2017). Instead, it is essential to adapt teaching to students' existing knowledge and skills, to help a learner form connections and acquire mastery – a sense of competence of being able to DO the skill (Bandura 2008) in a range of real-life situations. The extensive needs assessment work outlined in Chapters 1–3 ensures you have a great handle on where to start with learners to help them progress to the next stage of their learning.

Principle 2. Working in Partnership

Learning and behavioural theories have shown the importance of a collaborative and trusting learning space for learning and practice change, in which you (the trainer) and the learners are working in partnership (Felten 2013). Whether in adopting a new guideline at work, or making a change for their own health, people are the experts in knowing what will work for them in their own settings and are more likely to make lasting changes if motivation for change is internal, as evidenced by much research on self-determination theory (Ryan and Deci 2006) and motivational interviewing (Rollnick et al. 2010). The theory of self-determination recognises that people need autonomy and competence to drive change, whilst motivational interviewing is a communication style that encourages the person to become aware of their own behavioural discrepancies and actively confront their behaviour in an empathetic and accepting context. As trainers, we see our role as guides, facilitators and partners, offering a shared space and time and some ideas and choices to explore with different scenarios, to voice their own reasons for change and facilitate people building their own motivation, capability and opportunities for change. Building a collaborative and trusting training environment will be the foundation on which you then facilitate skills and knowledge development, and ultimately practice change, so it is worth thinking about how you will do this.

Principle 3. Interactive/Active Learning

Generally, evidence suggests we are more likely to remember information if we process it more deeply and it becomes 'meaningful' to us (Craik and Lockhard 1972), through opportunities to think about the information (e.g., through images or discussion), link it to previous knowledge or actively apply it to different situations. Also, as we will discuss in Chapters 2 and 3, health professional education also tends to have behavioural objectives – we aim to help learners make meaningful changes in their practice (rather than, for example, retain information to pass an exam). Research suggests that for skill development, learners need to build their confidence through repeated opportunities for practice and that those practices have to be long enough and of good quality (Ericsson and Harwell 2019).

For these reasons, the approaches suggested in this chapter aim to help trainers *start where the learners are, work in partnership* with learners through listening and enhancing their own motivations and abilities for change, and engaging them in *active learning* through evidence-based activities called Behaviour Change Techniques which encourage deeper processing of information and practicing new skills for use in their real-life practice.

Sometimes educators are worried about using active or playful learning because, depending on the experience of the learners, this might be something they are not used to. We have found that, after an initial surprise that the learning is not all instructional, people accept the interactive way of learning. When people engage in learning using different materials, it can help them to see things from new perspectives. It can make learning fun and more engaging. What we do know is that when learning is engaging it can increase the likelihood that people will learn and retain the information (Taylor and Hamdy 2013). Importantly as well, particularly for behaviour change, learning that is fun and playful can be remembered more easily and then can act as a prompt to remind people of what to do when back in their normal environments (Quillin and Thomas 2015).

Active learning can work best when introduced gently, building people's confidence in fun and play, such as the creation of name plates for introductions discussed below. Of all active learning techniques, practicing and rehearsing is vital. Haring et al.'s (1978) Learning Hierarchy is a useful reminder about the way we acquire new skills through repeated practice. At first, when we practice we are building up our accuracy (acquisition), then with time we become able to increase the speed we do the skill (fluency). However, more, real-life practice is needed to get us ready to recognise and use the skill in a wider range of settings (generalisation) before finally being able to adapt the skills for use in new challenging situations (adaptation).

Principle 4. Communication

As educators and trainers, you will know that how you communicate with your learners will have a big impact on their enjoyment and engagement. Communication is key to using behavioural science in education and training too. In Chapters 2 and 3, we discuss specifying the behaviours you want to change and exploring the influences on those behaviours. To do this effectively requires good communication within the education and training team and between the team and the learners. Techniques like reflective listening (listening to the person speaking and what they are also saying non-verbally, and reflecting this back to them) can be useful in this but is also itself a really useful teaching technique. When people speak, we can use this as an opportunity to use our own reflective listening to assist us to focus on what they have been saying but also to demonstrate the use of reflective listening to assist the learners in detecting how and when it can be used. You can demonstrate this, then highlight it and finally ask individuals to reflect – e.g. 'How might you have reflected what X has said? What did I say that you found useful, what might be a better way of reflecting that statement?'.

It is difficult to over-emphasise the importance of *listening* in building a collaborative training environment. Listening well and using reflective listening can be a powerful tool in your training repertoire. If you find that you are speaking more than 50% of the time, you are speaking too much. Asking questions that encourage individuals to think about their own behaviours can help to lead to discussion which you can then reflect. Much of your training should therefore be asking good open questions and then listening to the responses and reflecting these back.

Principle 5. A Collaborative Learning Environment

An essential task is to build a collaborative learning environment in which you create a sense of trust and develop connections between you, as the trainer, and the people you are training. This can be best achieved by listening well, encouraging the learners to talk and using reflective listening to demonstrate not only that you have heard, but also allowing the learner to hear their own words coming from you, thus helping to emphasise and amplify those words.

Building connections between the other learners is another rich contribution to the collaborative learning environment. Trainees will be able to support each other in learning. This is also valuable as together they can support each other. It can assist individuals to build confidence that they will not be isolated in undertaking this new behaviour. Other people will be doing it too and this can help to normalise the new behaviour.

Principle 6. Individual and Group Voices

Collecting the voices of the individual learners can be done in many different ways. To change the dynamics of any training, consider different groupings in which people will talk and exchange thoughts. Mix opportunities for discussion: in small groups, the whole group, in pairs or individual input. Not only will this help to alter the energy in the room, but it provides opportunities for people to hear the voices of others, avoids the domination of a handful of voices and supports those who feel less comfortable speaking out individually.

There will always be people in your group who feel less comfortable to speak out so it is important to give them easy ways of having their voices heard. Asking people to work in pairs or small groups and having one person (perhaps the more confident individual) reporting back can ensure that you are hearing all voices without putting anyone in an uncomfortable situation. You can use techniques whereby people demonstrate their thinking by holding up words or numbers, for example, placing numbers on a table and then asking people to pick up a number to show how confident they are. 'On a scale of 0–10, where 0 is not at all confident and 10 is extremely confident, pick up the number that shows how confident you are to overcome that problem'. (Note: we would only use this technique knowing the participants well enough to feel that they would not be uncomfortable demonstrating confidence levels to each other.) More generally, in training groups with difficult team dynamics or varying levels of knowledge, confidence and competence, the building blocks of your training, including a group agreement, are important to help ensure everyone can feel involved and included.

Principle 7. Time for Reflection

You will find many suggestions for different activities in this book. Activities on their own can be useful to help people engage with the learning; however, for activities to lead to learning, always ensure that there is time for reflection on that learning which strengthens the connection with the learning. For example, if you run an activity around role playing hand washing on a ward, be certain to reflect afterwards with the group. Good reflection-type questions might be: *What might be different in a real-life situation? What needs to happen for this to take place on a ward? What do you think happened in the role play that you hadn't thought about? If we were to repeat that role play, what might you change if it was you playing the XXX?*

In Chapters 2 and 3, we will describe in detail how to specify behaviours and explore the influences on those behaviours, which forms part of an overall 'theory of change'. In Chapter 4 we show how education and training activities can be selected that align with the theory of change, and in Chapter 5, we show how evaluation can be mapped directly onto the theory of change.

CHECK YOUR UNDERSTANDING AND REFLECT

1. Does the evidence support the idea that if someone knows how and can demonstrate doing something, they will do it accurately and routinely in real life?
2. What are some of the benefits of efforts such as the Behaviour Change Technique Taxonomy, to develop a shared language of the active ingredients of behaviour change interventions?
3. According to the COM-B framework, what are three kinds of influences on behaviour?
4. What can be the result of focusing only on improving capability when designing a new training course?
5. What are some of the main ways we can establish a collaborative learning environment during CPD courses?
6. What kinds of activities do you personally engage in for your own CPD?
7. What are some challenging training situations that you've experienced?

USEFUL LINKS AND FURTHER READING

Behavioural Theories and Types of Behaviours

http://www.behaviourchangetheories.com

Patey, A.M., Fontaine, G., Francis, J.J., McCleary, N., Presseau, J., and Grimshaw, J.M. (2022). Healthcare professional behaviour: health impact, prevalence of evidence-based behaviours, correlates and interventions. *Psychology & Health*. doi: 10.1080/08870446.2022.2100887.

Dual Processing

Kahneman, D. (2011). *Thinking, Fast and Slow*. UK: Penguin Books Limited.

The Com-B Framework

Michie, S., Atkins, L., and West, R. (2014) *The Behaviour Change Wheel: A Guide to Designing Interventions*. London, UK: Silverback Publishing.

http://www.behaviourchangewheel.com

Prime Theory and Other Briefings on Behaviour Change

https://www.unlockingbehaviourchange.com

https://www.hcpc-uk.org/cpd (2022)

REFERENCES

Bandura, A. (2008). An agentic perspective on positive psychology. In: *Praeger Perspectives. Positive Psychology: Exploring the Best in People*, 1 (ed. S.J. Lopez), 167–196. Westport, CT: Praeger Publishers/Greenwood Publishing Group.

Brown, C.A., Belfield, C.R., and Field, S.J. (2002). Cost effectiveness of continuing professional development in health care: a critical review of the evidence. *BMJ* 324 (7338): 652–655. 10.1136/bmj.324.7338.652.

Cilliers, F., Schuwirth, L., and van der Vleuten, C. (2015). Health Behaviour theories: a conceptual lens to explore behaviour change. In: *Researching Medical Education* (ed. J. Cleland and S.J. Durning), 141–154. Wiley-Blackwell. 10.1002/9781118838983.ch13.

Craik, F.I.M. and Lockhard, R.S. (1972). Levels of processing: a framework for memory research. *Journal of Verbal Learning and Verbal Behaviour* 11 (6): 671–684. 10.1016/S0022-5371(72)80001-X.

Cruess, R.L., Cruess, S.R., and Steinert, Y. (2016). Amending Miller's pyramid to include professional identity formation. *Academic Medicine* 91 (2): 180–185.

Eccles, M.P., Grimshaw, J.M., MacLennan, G., Bonetti, D., Glidewell, L., Pitts, N.B., Steen, N., Thomas, R., Walker, A., and Johnston, M. (2012). Explaining clinical behaviors using multiple theoretical models. *Implementation Science* 7: 99. 10.1186/1748-5908-7-99.

Ericsson, K.A. and Harwell, K.W. (2019). Deliberate practice and proposed limits on the effects of practice on the acquisition of expert performance: why the original definition matters and recommendations for future research. *Frontiers in Psychology* 10: 2396. 10.3389/fpsyg.2019.02396.

Evans, J.S.B.T. (2008). Dual-processing accounts of reasoning, judgment, and social cognition. *Annual Review of Psychology* 59: 255–278. 10.1146/annurev. psych.59.103006.093629.

Felten, P. (2013). Principles of good practice in SoTL. *Teaching and Learning Inquiry* 1 (1): 121–125. 10.20343/teachlearninqu.1.1.121.

Forsetlund, L., O'Brien, M.A., Forsén, L., Mwai, L., Reinar, L.M., Okwen, M.P., ... Rose, C.J. (2021). Continuing education meetings and workshops: effects on professional practice and healthcare outcomes. *Cochrane Database of Systematic Reviews.* Issue 9. Art. No.: CD003030 (DOI: https://doi. org/10.1002/14651858.CD003030.pub3).

Haring, N.G., Lovitt, T.C., Eaton, M.D., and Hansen, C.L. (1978). *The Fourth R: Research in the Classroom.* Columbus, OH: Charles E. Merrill Publishing Co.

Health and Care Professions Council (2022) Continuing professional development (CPD). Available at https://www.hcpc-uk.org/cpd/ (Accessed: 16th September 2022).

Kahneman, D. (2011). *Thinking, Fast and Slow.* Farrar: Straus and Giroux.

Karas, M., Sheen, N.J., North, R.V., Ryan, B., and Bullock, A. (2020). Continuing professional development requirements for UK health professionals: a scoping review. *BMJ Open* 10 (3): e032781. https://doi.org/10.1136/bmjopen-2019-03278.

Kirschner, P.A. (2017). Stop propagating the learning styles myth. *Computers & Education* 106: 166–171. 10.1016/j.compedu.2016.12.006.

Légaré, F., Freitas, A., Thompson-Leduc, P., Borduas, F., Lucioni, F., Boucher, A., Witteman, H.O., and Jacques, A. (2015). The majority of accredited continuing professional development activities do not target clinical behaviour change. *Academic Medicine* 90 (2): 197–202. doi: 10.1097/ACM.0000000000000543.

Luangasanatip, N., Hongsuwan, M., Limmathurotsakul, D., Lubell, Y., Lee, A.S., Harbarth, S., Day, N.P.J., Graves, N., and Cooper, B.S. (2015). Comparative efficacy of interventions to promotehand hygiene in hospital: systematic review and network meta-analysis. *BMJ* 351: h3728. 10.1136/bmj.h3728.

McCay, L. (2015). Emotional motivators might improve hand hygiene among healthcare workers. *BMJ* 351: h3968.

Michie, S., Johnston, M., Abraham, C., Lawton, R., Parker, D., and Walker, A. (2005). Making psychological theory useful for implementing evidence based practice: a consensus approach. *Quality and Safety in Health Care* 14 (1): 26–33. 10.1136/qshc.2004.011155.

Michie, S., Richardson, M., Johnston, M., Abraham, C., Francis, J., Hardeman, W., Eccles, M.P., Cane, K., and Wood, C.E. (2013). The behavior change technique taxonomy (v1) of 93 hierarchically clustered techniques: building an international consensus for the reporting of behavior change interventions. *Annals of Behavioural Medicine* 46 (1): 81–95. 10.1007/s12160-013-9486-6.

Michie, S., van Stralen, M.M., and West, R. (2011). The behaviour change wheel: a new method for characterising and designing behaviour change interventions. *Implementation Science* 6: 42. 10.1186/1748-5908-6-42.

Michie, S., West, R., Campbell, R., Brown, J., and Gainforth, G. (2014). *ABC of Behaviour Change Theories*. Silverback Pubishing. ISBN: 978-1-912141-01-2.

Miller, G.E. (1990). The assessment of clinical skills/competence/performance. *Academic Medicine* 65 (9): S63–7.

Pearson, E., Byrne-Davis, L., Bull, E., and Hart, J. (2020). Behavior change techniques in health professional training: developing a coding tool. *Translational Behavioral Medicine* 10 (1): 96–102. 10.1093/tbm/iby125.

Peck, C., McCall, M., McLaren, B., and Rotem, T. (2000). Continuing medical education and continuing professional development: international comparisons. *BMJ* 320 (7232): 432–435. 10.1136/bmj.320.7232.432.

Presseau, J., Johnston, M., Heponiemi, T., Elovainio, M., Francis, J.J., Eccles, M.P., Steen, N., Hrisos, S., Stamp, E., Grimshaw, J.M., Hawthorne, G., and Sniehotta, F.F. (2014). Reflective and automatic processes in health care professional behaviour: a dual process model tested across multiple behaviours. *Annals of Behavioural Medicine* 48 (3): 347–358. 10.1007/s12160-014-9609-8.

Qullin, K & Thomas, S. (2015) Drawing to learn: A framework for using drawings to promote model-based reasoning in biology. *CBE – Life Sciences Education* 14: 1–6.

Rollnick, S., Butler, C.C., Kinnersley, P., Gregory, J., and Mash, B. (2010 Motivational interviewing. BMJ 340: c1900 .https://doi.org/10.1136/bmj.c1900.

Ryan, R.M. and Deci, E.L. (2006). Self-regulation and the problem of human autonomy: does psychology need choice, self-determination, and will? *Journal of Personality* 74: 1557–1585. 10.1111/j.1467-6494.2006.00420.x.

Taylor, D.C.M. and Hamdy, H. (2013). Adult learning theories: implications for learning and teaching in medical education: AMEE Guide No. 83. *Medical Teacher* 35 (11): e1561–e1572. 10.3109/0142159X.2013.828153.

Thaler, R.H. and Sunstein, C.R. (2021). *Nudge: The Final Edition.* UK: Penguin Random House.

West, R. and Brown, J. (2014). *Theory of Addiction.* Oxford, UK: Wiley.

World Health Organisation. (2022). *Global Competency and Outcomes Framework for Universal Health Coverage.* ISBN: 978 92 4 003466 2. Licence CC BY-NC-SA 3.0 IGO

Yoong, S.L., Hall, A., Stacey, F., Grady, A., Sutherland, R., Wyse, R., Anderson, A., Nathan, N., and Wolfenden, L. (2020). Nudge strategies to improve health-care providers' implementation of evidence-based guidelines, policies and practices: a systematic review of trials included within Cochrane systematic reviews. *Implementation Science* 15 (1): 50. 10.1186/s13012-020-01011-0.

CHAPTER 2

Defining the Behaviours That You Want to Change

Learning Points

- It can be difficult to 'think behaviourally'; it is unusual for courses to define specific behaviours
- The process of defining behaviours can be a good way of stakeholders making their own assumptions explicit
- Many behaviours, involving many people, are usually changed to make a beneficial final outcome
- Specify *who* needs to do *what*, *how*, *to* or *with whom*, *when* and *where*
- Create a theory of change that links training, influences on behaviour, behaviours and outcomes

Training to Change Practice: Behavioural Science to Develop Effective Health Professional Education, First Edition. Jo Hart, Lucie Byrne-Davis, Wendy Maltinsky, and Eleanor Bull. © 2023 John Wiley & Sons Ltd. Published 2023 by John Wiley & Sons Ltd.

INTRODUCTION

We start by thinking about what we want to achieve with our training. In this chapter, we will take you beyond thinking of what the learner will learn to what we hope they might *do* differently afterwards, as they return to their own practice.

Most educators will be familiar with the concept of setting intended learning outcomes. These typically describe what the learner will know and/ or be able to do after completion of the activities. Intended learning outcomes have become the bedrock of most education, implementing the paradigm of learning called 'outcomes based education' (Albanese et al. 2008). Intended learning outcomes are distinct from the *aims* of the education, which might be broader than the learners themselves knowing more and might include aims such as improving patient outcomes or experience. The *objectives* of the education are then more specific details about how you propose your education might lead to you realising the aims. As such, aims and objectives are both focused on the educator, i.e. what they think, and they intend. Intended learning outcomes are focused on the learner, i.e. how we expect them to have changed after participating in the activities.

What an individual knows and can do can usefully be thought of as their competency or capability. In much health professional education, competency-based education is the norm. For people who are not yet practicing in their health profession, it makes sense that education is focused on developing capability or competency in particular skills. Undoubtedly, we want health professionals who are capable of doing the important tasks that make up their roles. In Chapter 1 we summarised some of the behavioural science evidence reminding us that capability is only one influence on our behaviour – just because we can do something, doesn't mean we will! What is also clear is that acting on our capabilities sometimes involves us doing several things differently, i.e. there are multiple behaviours that add up to make any person's role. With this in mind, it is important that as health professional educators you are thinking not only about an individual's capability but also their motivation to change and the opportunities they have to change all the behaviours that make up a new guideline or service development.

Going beyond intended learning outcomes means we automatically start to take our focus out of the classroom, back into environments where our learners will try their new ideas and skills. These are going to often be tricky to use in real-life practice and thinking of where we want them to head for helps us stay on track. Knowing where we're aiming also helps us all know if we've got there and explore what helped and got in the way. They also serve as a form of behavioural commitment for both trainers and learners, setting out what each party can hope for and expect.

DEVELOPING A THEORY OF CHANGE

A theory of change links activities to changes that are expected to lead to desired outcomes (Vogel 2012). Sometimes, we call this setting out the programme logic, because it is the logical steps between where we are now, what we are going to do and where we think that will take us. A theory of change, with added behavioural science, means that we also spell out what we expect our CPD to do to the learners' capabilities, opportunities and motivations. For CPD, a theory of change will link the education activities through changes expected in the learner to changes expected in the practices of the learner and perhaps to improved patient or other higher-level outcomes.

Developing a theory of change is enlightening and gives you a way to evaluate your CPD. The process, if done with your team and perhaps even some other stakeholders, allows you to put your CPD into the context of your learners. It will ask you to think about what you expect to change in your learners after they have done your CPD and then what you expect them to do differently afterwards. We like to develop a theory of change through a series of workshops (see Tips and examples box), in which we discuss and agree on the aims of the CPD in terms of three levels of outcome: patient/clinical outcome; changes in the practice of the health professionals; changes in the capability, opportunity and motivation of the health professionals. We then ask the question, what parts of your CPD are intending to address these changes in capability, opportunity, motivation and practice.

Tips and examples

Workshop 1: Specifying outcomes and indicators

- Specify what would happen if your CPD was to be successful. You can get people to do this individually and then discuss, or you can get them to discuss in groups or altogether.
- Once the group have agreed what would happen, then ask them to think about how they would know if those things had happened. It is good practice to have outcomes that can be measured in some way (see Chapter 5 for evaluation).

Workshop 2: Developing a pathway to change

- Ask who needs to what differently to reach each outcome and make sure these are specific (see this chapter).
- Ask what needs to change for the people identified to do the behaviours you have specified. You can usefully prompt by thinking of capability, opportunity and motivation here. If you don't know and you have time, you can do some further work in exploring influences (see Chapter 3).

Workshop 3: Mapping your CPD to the pathway

- Take each outcome and pathway in turn and ask the question: what in our CPD addresses this?

Draft a theory of change connecting outcomes, activities and pathways to change and send around the stakeholder group and encourage further discussion as appropriate.

Finalise and agree your CPD theory of change.

INTENDED BEHAVIOURAL OUTCOMES (IBOs)

It is important to detail each of the *intended behavioural outcomes (IBOs)* of the education and training activities. These IBOs detail what you expect the health professional *to do* or *not to do* when they return to work after the education and training.

When listing the IBOs, take care to specify all aspects of the behaviour. Research has identified these aspects as action, actor, context, target and time (AACTT) (Presseau et al. 2019) but we think of these as WHO needs to do WHAT, HOW, WITH WHOM, WHEN and WHERE.

Action: WHAT and HOW is the action being performed?

Actor: WHO is doing the behaviour (e.g., nurse, doctor, family member)

Context: WHERE is the behaviour being performed?

Target: WITH WHOM is the behaviour performed, e.g., patient or colleague?

Time: WHEN is the behaviour being performed, e.g., after admission, before touching a patient?

IBOs can include being clear about the things that we would like people to start, stop and continue doing in their practice. 'Continue' might also mean changing slightly, altering **how** they might do this. For example, *'continue to wash hands but increase from 1 minute to 2 minutes'*.

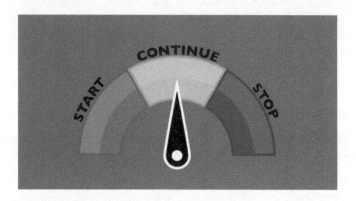

Tips and examples

It might help, to construct a sentence that specifies each IBO. For example, if you were targeting the cleaning of a woman's back prior to spinal anaesthesia during caesarean section, you might have as an IBO:

The individual responsible for anaesthesia (WHO) will clean each woman's back (WHAT WITH WHOM) with the appropriate equipment (HOW) in the operating room (WHERE) before any contact is made between scalpel and back (WHEN).

If you were trying to reduce antibiotic prescribing in primary care centres for upper respiratory tract infection you might have as an IBO:

The prescriber (WHO) in the primary care centre (WHERE) will counsel the patient, using behaviour change communication (HOW) and not prescribe antibiotics (WHAT) to a patient with an upper respiratory tract infection but no symptoms indicating bacterial infection (WITH WHOM) during a consultation (WHEN).

HOW TO DEVELOP IBOs

Our research has shown that training interventions often try to change around 50 behaviours, although we have seen up to around 200 in some courses. It would be impossible to create IBOs for each of these. Rather, we suggest that the development team decide which ones are the most important to target. The importance you place on the targeted behaviours might be because they are the hardest behaviours to change, or because they are the behaviours that would have the most impact if changed or even because they were the easiest to change and would therefore bring the most success. In fact, there are lots of reasons why you might choose specific behaviours on which to focus. There are no right or wrong reasons but doing this deliberately ensures that you are working towards achieving your goals of training.

Our experience has shown that specifying IBOs and creating specific behavioural definition statements is not easy for project teams. Often people talk about improved staff confidence, team culture or client outcomes as if they are IBOs (Bull et al. 2019a, b). We might need to ask more questions to understand where the IBOs lie, for instance 'And what would we be doing differently to achieve these better outcomes?' 'What could we see each other doing or not doing if we had more confidence as a team?' 'What would a good team culture look like?' Time spent building our understanding through our logic model, can really help us unroll a knotty problem and find our IBOs. Some IBOs may also be tricky as they relate to effective clinical decision-making – which includes many skills but few overtly observable behaviours (NHS Education for Scotland 2013). In this case, IBOs may relate to behaviours that help a clinician come to a good decision (e.g., the kind of assessment a clinician does, listening skills to gather cues, use of records and lab results, listening to own experience and 'gut feelings') and the behaviours following the decision (e.g., performing actions in a timely way, communicating with others about the actions, reviewing and checking the outcomes of the decision).

There are several ways of developing IBOs. In our experience, the easiest method is for the whole team to meet (either online or in person) for a group discussion/workshop. Whilst this might be easier if the meeting is facilitated by a behavioural scientist or someone who is experienced in facilitation and understands about behavioural specification, it is perfectly possible to learn these skills and put them into practice. Another benefit of holding a team meeting like this is that the team might not have sat down before and identified crucial behaviours within job roles. Having a group discussion about this can identify misunderstandings or differences of opinion that can then lead to better group cohesion. This can form part of the development of your theory of change.

Sometimes IBOs need to be shaped over time – with an 'ideas board' on a ward where people can add IBOs on post it notes. This may be important especially if the topic is sensitive and there are many possible routes to change. In one ward we worked in where two teams had been merged together, resulting in what they described as 'cultural problems', this led to the team self-generating many ideas for changes over several weeks, which in itself started to turn the conversation around towards positive change (Bull et al. 2019a).

Tips and examples: Topic guide and cues for a behavioural specification focus group

The key outcomes for the training

Encourage the team to list things they want to achieve by doing the training (they might have these already in another form, e.g. a log frame) and note these on a flipchart/white board/online whiteboard. Prompt to think about outcomes for everyone – staff, patients, public or other stakeholders.

Taking each outcome in turn, can you think about what the health professionals would have to do if that outcome was to happen?

Take outcomes one at a time, ask for practices. If teams give knowledge, skills, attitudes, ask them to restate these as behaviours. It helps to describe behaviours and things you can see people doing or not doing.

For each practice, let's spell out who needs to do what, when, where, when, to whom and how

Create 'specification' statements for each behaviour.

WHAT DOES THE EVIDENCE SAY?

Specifying behaviours is a consensus-type activity. There are multiple papers written about consensus activities, with perhaps the most common being a Delphi Study. A Delphi Study is a series of surveys, usually online, that seek to gain consensus on an issue. In the case of Delphi studies for generating intended behavioural outcomes, the first survey would ask people to think of behaviours that they think the programme is aiming to influence. The second survey would then present these results back to the participants and then there would be some sort of selection or ranking, with comments. The third survey would then present back these results and so on, until consensus is reached, or you reach a predefined stopping point. Delphi studies have been used a lot in the development of core outcome sets for effectiveness trials of treatments and interventions in health care. The main benefits are that they are low cost and that they allow people to contribute equally, regardless of how confident they feel speaking or discussing in a group.

We have found that it is quite hard to get consensus for behaviours targeted by education and training programmes using the Delphi method only. We find that the act of having discussions helps people to come to a shared understanding. If you thought that some people would be disadvantaged by using a talking method alone, then it would be possible to do a hybrid of workshop and Delphi. For this, it would be good to have an initial workshop in which the ideas around behaviours and behaviour change were discussed before moving into an online Delphi. For more reading about Delphi studies, there are some good resources from Involve and the COMET initiative (see useful links).

CHOOSING THE IBOs ON WHICH TO FOCUS

It is not unusual for courses to have 50 or more IBOs. It can be difficult to change behaviours and partly this is due to the mental load of thinking about the behaviour and controlling yourself. It is possible then that asking your learners to change many behaviours might overload them such that they don't change at all, although some of the many IBOs might be interlinked or they might be IBOs for different members of the team. It is important, though, if you are going to explore the influences on your IBOs or try to change them in your training, to select a handful (perhaps between 5 and 10) on which to focus. These could be the IBOs that would have the most impact in terms of patient outcomes. They might be the ones that are easiest to change. Many CPD courses go through multiple rounds, with people doing them more than once over a period of time. It is possible, therefore, to use the information on behavioural influences to target different IBOs in different iterations of your training programme. This doesn't mean that you can't mention the other changes in your CPD, of course, but they might form less of a part whilst you are focusing on the key behaviours.

WHOSE IBOs ARE THEY?

As trainers, it is important to reflect on our roles and how attached we are to our training IBOs. The IBOs may feel like 'ours' – if we have designed a training course to address what feels an important practice issue. They may be 'come from above', and be a change decided on by senior managers or decreed by local or national guidelines. Or they may be IBOs the team have selected, or asked for your help implementing, as above. This might be important to discuss openly and honestly with busy healthcare practitioner colleagues as it impacts on motivation (the M of COM) and can affect engagement in training courses from the start. We often find new guidelines or initiatives appear at first glance to involve ever-increasing tasks on the to-do list. This quite rightly leads practitioners to ask 'ok so if I'm going to also do this, what do you want me to stop doing?!' A deeper dive into guidelines or service contracts may identify areas where time can be saved by other 'stop' practice changes, which can enhance motivation to engage in training.

At times, we may find our role might involve being an advocate for 'change fatigued' or even burned-out practitioners. IBO specification may lead to (with a group's permission) you feeding back concerns a group has about what seem like values-incongruent or impossible IBOs to managers and other service leads. As a trainer, it can be anxiety-provoking, but ultimately most useful to have compassionate conversations with managers where you believe training is not the right intervention for a healthcare team.

CHECK YOUR UNDERSTANDING

1. Why is it useful to think about your Intended Behavioural Outcomes when starting to plan education and training?
2. What does AACTT stand for when specifying behaviours?
3. Think back to the last training course where you were a learner. What were some of its main Intended Behavioural Outcomes: things the trainers hoped you would start, stop or continue doing in your work practice after attending?
4. Thinking about the next CPD training course you are leading and using what you've learnt in this chapter, have a go at designing some IBOs for the participants in your training.

USEFUL LINKS AND FURTHER READING

Developing A Theory of Change

COMET Initiative, which is a network for people interested in the development and application of core outcome sets. https://www.comet-initiative.org/assets/downloads/Delphi%20plain%20language%20summary%20for%20COMET%20website.pdf.

The Community Builder's Approach to Theory of Change, The Aspen Institute. https://www.theoryofchange.org/pdf/TOC_fac_guide.pdf.

Involve. https://www.involve.org.uk/resources/methods/delphi-survey.

REFERENCES

Albanese, M.A., Mejicano, G., Mullan, P., Kokotailo, P., and Gruppen, L. (2008). Defining characteristics of educational competencies. *Medical Education* 42: 248–255.

Bull ER, Byrne-Davis LMT, Swift J, Baxter K, McLauchlan N, Hart JK. Exploring what teams perceive by 'culture' *when implementing new models of care. Int J Qual Health Care.* 2019a Jul 1;31(6):492–494. doi: 10.1093/intqhc/mzy200. PMID: 30256985.

Bull ER, Hart JK, Swift J, Baxter K, McLauchlan N, Joseph S, Byrne-Davis LMT. An organisational participatory research study of the feasibility of the behaviour change wheel to support clinical teams implementing new models of care. BMC Health Serv Res. 2019b Feb 4;19(1):97. doi: 10.1186/s12913-019-3885-8 PMID: 30717764; PMCID: PMC6360652.

NHS Education for Scotland. (2013). Clinical decision making. https://www.effectivepractitioner.nes.scot.nhs.uk/clinical-practice/clinical-decision-making.aspx (accessed 4 July 2022).

Presseau, J., McCleary, N., Lorencatto, F. et al. (2019). Action, actor, context, target, time (AACTT): a framework for specifying behaviour. *Implementation Science* 14: 102.

Vogel, I. (2012). *Review of the Use of Theory of Change in International Development.* London: UK Department of International Development.

CHAPTER 3

Exploring the Influences on Behaviours

Learning Points

- Capability, motivation and opportunity (COM) are part of a helpful framework for understanding influences on practice
- Exploring COM before developing education and training can help to pitch sessions
- If it is not possible to explore COM before education and training, you can explore these influences during the education and training

As we outlined in Chapter 1, there are multiple factors that will influence how someone practices, behaves or acts. This includes the competency and capability of the learner in the particular skill or behaviour, but there are many other influences. If we are trying to influence practice with our education and training, therefore, we need to spend time learning what these

Training to Change Practice: Behavioural Science to Develop Effective Health Professional Education, First Edition. Jo Hart, Lucie Byrne-Davis, Wendy Maltinsky, and Eleanor Bull. © 2023 John Wiley & Sons Ltd. Published 2023 by John Wiley & Sons Ltd.

influences are so that we can develop activities that address crucial barriers and use facilitators.

INFLUENCES ON PRACTICE

There are a range of factors that will influence whether someone does each of the IBOs in practice. As outlined in Chapter 1, these can be usefully summarised as capability, opportunity and motivation (Michie et al. 2011, see Figure 3).

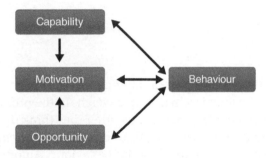

FIGURE 3   The COM-B framework (Michie et al. 2011/Springer Nature/CC BY 2.0).

Capability

Capability is both physical and psychological which are skills and knowledge respectively.

Tips and examples

Typical capability statements include:
I know it
I know how to do it
I know when to do it
I have the mental space to do it

Opportunity

Opportunity is both physical and social. Physical opportunity covers things like time and equipment and colleagues to do tasks with or for you. Social opportunity is best summarised as 'the way we do things round here' and is sometimes known as culture, peer pressure or hidden curriculum.

Tips and examples

Typical opportunity statements include:
I have everything I need to do it
People whose opinion I care about think I should do it
I have enough time to do this
The computer system allows me to do this
My manager approves of me doing this
Colleagues think this is a good idea

Motivation

Motivation is both reflective and automatic.

Reflective motivation is when people weigh up the pros and cons of the behaviour and will include things like whether they think the behaviour will lead to a good end point, whether the behaviour is difficult or easy and whether they feel in control of doing the behaviour. Automatic motivation includes impulses to carry out the behaviour and things like habit and conditioning (learning over time, repeat experiences).

Tips and examples

Typical motivation statements include:
On balance I think it is a good idea
It is part of my usual practice
I just do it without really thinking too much about it

HOW TO EXPLORE INFLUENCES ON EACH IBO

It is important, when thinking about what to include in education and training, to explore the capability, opportunity and motivation of each IBO with a sample of the population of those who are expected to do each behaviour. This is ideally done before developing the education and training, but is not always feasible. Remember that COM is about barriers to behaviours but also about facilitators to behaviours.

BEFORE DEVELOPING CPD

Sometimes, it will be possible to gather the information you need on the COMs of each IBO through a series of interviews or focus groups or observations of practice before you plan your CPD. You can use questionnaires and often educators use a pre-course needs assessment or pre-course evaluation. To increase the behavioural focus, you can ask different questions and two questionnaires in particular have been developed to assess the COM around specific behaviours (Keyworth et al. 2020) and even more granular influences on behaviour (Huijg et al. 2014) (see Further Reading).

If you are talking to people directly, remember to use all the good communication skills that you know. These are the same as the skills that help us to talk to patients and to run good training courses.

Tips and examples

Active listening: Eye contact, nodding, saying 'go on' 'mmm', creating rapport, using pauses, being/looking interested, being genuine

Non-verbal components of listening: Eye contact, posture, gestures, facial expressions, use of voice (tone, timing, emphasis on certain words, vocalisations other than words)

Open and closed questions: Open questions (e.g., how are you feeling?) are broad and require more than a one or two word answer. They often begin with: what, why, when, how, where, who? Closed questions (e.g., are you feeling ill?) limit the possible answers to 'yes', 'no' or a one-word answer.

Reflective skills:

- Reflection (saying back to someone all or part of what they have just said) may help them to carry on and expand.
- Paraphrasing (rephrasing in your own words what someone has just said) may verify your understanding and help them to carry on or expand further.
- Silence allows people time to think about what they have said and allow you time to plan the next stage.
- Summarising allows checking and reviewing, keeps people on track if they are wandering off subject, lets someone know you have been listening, helps to close an interaction.

Building rapport:

- Setting: Try to make the person feel at ease by getting the setting right – e.g., if you are in their home, ask which chair they would like you to sit in; appropriate positioning of chairs (at a comfortable angle); quiet and private environment.
- Eye level: Try to be at the same eye level as the person.
- Introduce yourself: full name and role.
- Give time and attention to the person.
- Notice the person's method of self-expression (minimal cues, e.g. what's said and what's not said, pace and tone of voice, posture, eye contact).
- It is sometimes helpful to try to match some of the minimal cues, without being patronising.
- Avoid inappropriate use of jargon and aim to match your vocabulary to that of the person. Avoid talking down to the person.

It is useful to think who is the most appropriate person or people to do this information gathering. Sometimes, it is useful to be an independent 'naïve' interviewer/observer because you can ask questions that would seem ignorant or strange coming from a health professional working in that field. Sometimes, people are worried about why the independent person is asking the questions and then it might be useful to have a fellow health professional exploring these barriers and facilitators. In work, where there is a power differential, e.g., where the interviewer/observer is from a high-income country and the health professionals from a low-income country (or where the former is senior and the latter junior) this can influence how comfortable people are to talk about difficulties.

Be aware that health professionals might feel more inhibited talking about different types of barriers. In recent work, we found that opportunity and time might seem more acceptable to discuss as barriers, rather than saying that you don't agree with the policy or are suspicious of the guidelines (Whittenbury et al. 2022). GPs have been found to use the concept of being short of time when discussing barriers to recruitment into clinical trials, although further exploration indicated that this was more an issue of prioritisation (Salmon et al. 2007).

Sometimes, it won't be possible to conduct a series of interviews or focus groups systematically, or to do enough interviews that you capture the full range of views. Be prepared to have ad hoc conversations with health professionals that you meet, and (with appropriate permissions from them) make some field notes. You might also observe people practicing and you should make use of these observations to comment on COM in your field notes.

Tips and examples

Remember to introduce the specific behaviour you are collecting information about. Explain that you want to understand what might help someone do that behaviour or what gets in the way. Allow conversation to flow but try to ask some open questions that specifically address capability, opportunity and motivation.

Is there anything that would get in the way of you doing that? (general)

When you are able to do that? What is it that helps? (general)

What do you think you need to know if you are going to do that? (psychological capability)

What skills do you think you need if you are going to do that? (physical capability)

What do other people think about you doing that? (social or physical opportunity)

What do you need if you are going to do that (prompt, e.g., time, equipment, other resources, other people)? (physical opportunity)

What do you think people at work think about you doing that (prompt patients, colleagues) or what would they think if you started doing it? (social opportunity)

It is important for you to do that? (reflective motivation)

How easy is it for you to do that? (reflective motivation)

Do you think it is part of your role to do that? (reflective motivation)

Do you think that helps patients? (reflective motivation)

Do you do this automatically? (automatic motivation)

DURING CPD

If you are unable to explore behavioural influences fully for each IBO, then you can explore COM as part of the training by including activities in which learners and facilitators discuss barriers and enablers. See Chapter 4.

CHECK YOUR UNDERSTANDING AND REFLECT

1. What are some of the main ways we can explore influences on colleagues' practices?
2. What kinds of questions best help elicit influences, during focus groups, interviews or ad hoc conversations?
3. What role, organisational position, skills or experience do you think is needed to conduct exploring of influences and why?
4. If a midwife told you she thinks the behaviour of 'having health promoting conversations with pregnant mums about physical activity' is a good idea, but she always forgets to do this, which kind of barrier is this according to the COM-B Framework?
5. Why might some barriers be more socially acceptable for colleagues to talk about than others?

FURTHER READING

More About Exploring Influences on Behaviour

Chapter 1 of Michie, S., Atkins, L., and West, R. (2014). *The Behaviour Change Wheel: A Guide to Designing Interventions*. London: Silverback Publishing.

REFERENCES

Huijg, J.M., Gebhardt, W.A., Dusseldorp, E., Verheijden, M.W., van der Zouwe, N., Middelkoop, B.J., and Crone, M.R. (2014). Measuring determinants of implementation behavior: psychometric properties of a questionnaire based on the theoretical domains framework. *Implementation Science* 9: 33. doi: 10.1186/1748-5908-9-33.

Keyworth, C., Epton, T., Goldthorpe, J., Calam, R., and Armitage, C.J. (2020 September). Acceptability, reliability, and validity of a brief measure of capabilities, opportunities, and motivations ("COM-B"). *British Journal of Health Psychology* 25 (3): 474–501. doi: 10.1111/bjhp.12417. Epub 2020 Apr 20. PMID: 32314500.

Michie, S., van Stralen, M.M., and West, R. (2011). The behaviour change wheel: a new method for characterising and designing behaviour change interventions. *Implementation Science* 6: 42.

Salmon, P., Peters, S., Rogers, A., Gask, L., Clifford, R., Iredale, W., Dowrick, C., and Morriss, R. (2007). Peering through the barriers in GPs' explanations for declining to participate in research: the role of professional autonomy and the economy of time. *Family Practice* 24 (3): 269–275.

Whittenbury, K., Kroll, L., Dubicka, B., and Bull, E.R. (2022). Exploring barriers and facilitators for mental health professionals delivering behavioural activation to young people with depression: qualitative study using the Theoretical Domains Framework. *BJPsych Open* 8 (2):1–11.

CHAPTER 4

Developing CPD to Change Behaviour

Learning Points

- CPD contains active ingredients which aim to change our learners' practice. These are called behaviour change techniques
- You can develop training with techniques to both target barriers to change and work with facilitators to change
- Techniques in training to support change can target capability, opportunity, motivation or a combination and active learning approaches helps learning stick, making change more likely

The earlier chapters have identified behaviours to change and the influences on those behaviours. Understanding these is vital in helping you decide your targets for change in education and training activities and enabling you to be able to measure if your training has changed practice. In this chapter, we

Training to Change Practice: Behavioural Science to Develop Effective Health Professional Education, First Edition. Jo Hart, Lucie Byrne-Davis, Wendy Maltinsky, and Eleanor Bull. © 2023 John Wiley & Sons Ltd. Published 2023 by John Wiley & Sons Ltd.

turn to the exciting and creative process of developing and delivering behaviourally informed and engaging training activities. We draw on our experiences as psychologists and educators as well as developments from the research fields of behavioural science and pedagogy in offering suggestions and approaches for you to think about as a training team.

THE ACTIVE INGREDIENTS OF BEHAVIOUR CHANGE ACTIVITIES

One of the key developments in behavioural science over the past decade has been to name and define active ingredients of our behaviour change interventions, known as behaviour change techniques. Every organised effort to change behaviour includes one or more behaviour change techniques: from a poster to encourage pregnant women to stop smoking to a training course to help trainee nurses to adopt good hand hygiene. In the UK, behavioural scientists developed the Behaviour Change Technique Taxonomy (Michie et al. 2013), a structured list of 93 BCTs, including techniques like facilitating 'goal setting' or giving 'information about health consequences' of a behaviour. For practitioners and educators, being able to name and describe the tools in our 'behaviour change toolbox' means we can more easily select the best ones for the training session or other activities which assist practitioners to change behaviours. BCTs change behaviour by enhancing motivation, capability, opportunity or a combination of these. From our research with health professional educators, we think around 43 BCTs are suitable for use in education and training (Pearson et al. 2018) which we focus on in this section.

REMINDER: WHAT IS COM-B AGAIN?

The COM-B model of behaviour summarises three interlinking factors that need to be present for any behaviour (B) to happen: capability (C), opportunity (O) and motivation (M). *Capability* is *psychological* and *physical*: a person's knowledge and skills to do the behaviour. *Opportunity* includes influential factors in the *physical* environment (e.g., time or equipment) or *social* environment (social pressures and support). *Motivation* includes both *reflective* attitudes and decision making, and *automatic* habits, routes and emotional responses that drive many of the things we do each day whilst on 'autopilot'. COM-B is at the heart of the Behaviour Change Wheel approach to designing behaviour change interventions (Michie et al. 2014). When individuals, groups or communities pin down behaviour(s) needing to change and have a good understanding of the main influences upon them, this helps them choose relevant training or other activities with helpful behaviour change techniques to support their change efforts.

BCTS AND COMMUNICATION SKILLS IN EDUCATION AND TRAINING

BCTs and communication skills can be found throughout education and training. This includes what the trainer says, asks or does (including simple prompts for group discussions), in audio/visual and written materials (including slides/handouts) and any resources given out (e.g., posters or equipment) for use back in work or study.

Tips and examples

Some examples of using BCTs and communication skills in your training:

Environmental Restructuring:
Create a poster to consider 'changing the environment': 'what's different poster'. Provide an activity which shows the same scene but in which there may be very slight changes, i.e. the placing of hand sanitiser in places where it might remind us to use it in contrast to obvious places where it might not be useful – in a cupboard or under a patient's bed etc. A 'spot the difference' poster can be a fun way of demonstrating how environmental restructuring assists with implementing a behaviour like using hand sanitiser

Habit:
To introduce the idea of 'automatic motivation', ask people how they arrived at the session and for them to describe their journey. Many will not remember because we tend to go onto automatic pilot when we travel to work. This is a good opportunity to talk about all sorts of automatic behaviours. We might demonstrate how we as trainers we are guided by automatic motivation too, and ask learners to spot our habits during the session. Raising awareness of habits and routines helps us in our efforts to change those we are trying to erode as well as those we are trying to create.

Many experienced training facilitators skilfully and automatically use BCTs to great effect without thinking about the theories and methods of behaviour change. However, when designing a new course from scratch, it can be useful to follow a structured process which helps us to match IBOs and BCTs which strengthen capability, opportunity and/or motivation. To help people with this process, we brought together health psychologists and educators to develop Cards for Change – 45 ideas for training activities which put BCTs into action, see the 'Cards for Change' section at the end of the book (Byrne-Davis et al. 2022).

BCTs are used here in terms of how we make training engaging and impactful, but we can also find ourselves teaching our learners to use the same BCTs with others in their practice (e.g., managers with teams, or practitioners with members of the public). For an example of BCTs used at both levels, please see Bull and Dale (2021).

HOW TO DEVELOP YOUR TRAINING ACTIVITIES

Take each of your IBOs in turn (see Chapter 2). Remind yourself of the influences on each IBO (Chapter 3) for example what capability, opportunity or motivation barriers are getting in the way of your learners *doing* the desired practices? If you haven't had chance already, you may need to ask learners about this as one of the first activities of the training. This could involve inviting the group to write down barriers and facilitators to doing certain practices on a post-it note assembled in one place, or using an online programme such as Padlet for virtual training and posting their ideas of the barriers and facilitators there. In an e-learning training, this might include activities where people could 'click' on characters to reveal 'common thoughts' about the topic in question which they may relate to and a prompt to note down for themselves if they would add any others.

Now choose training activities incorporating BCTs that can address these challenges and opportunities.

Table 1 includes examples of how specific BCTs can be used in training activities that tie in with the psychological mechanisms behind capability, opportunity and motivation. This table draws on the Cards for Change, The Behaviour Change Wheel (Michie et al. 2014, pp. 284–289) and the Theory and Techniques Tool (see Further Reading). We expand on these for building capability, opportunity and motivation below. For more education and training activities see the 'Guides' section at the end of the book.

TABLE 1 Examples of how specific BCTs in training can relate to Capability, Opportunity and Motivation (COM).

BCT	Example training activities	Behavioural influences that might change					
		Capability		Opportunity		Motivation	
		Physical	Psychological	Physical	Social	Reflective	Automatic
Goal setting (behaviour)	State the behavioural aim, e.g. 'the goal of this session is to change the way you assess a critically ill patient'.					▓	
Information about health, social or environmental consequences	Include facts and figures and stories from real people about how things are better if the behaviour is changed. Ask learners to match facts and figures to find, e.g. the cost savings the health service could make if we all prescribed antibiotics in line with guidelines.				▓	▓	
Pros and cons	Ask learners to gather their ideas on the pros and cons of making a change to their practice.					▓	
Instruction on how to perform the behaviour and Demonstration of the behaviour	Demonstrate a skill, talking through how to do each step (you could use an acronym if there are several steps).	▓	▓				

Behavioural practice and rehearsal	Practice in groups of threes (practitioner, client and observer). This could be role play (with a scenario) or real play (an issue that is really affecting the 'client'). Ask learners to practice it enough times to feel like an 'over-rehearsal': so they can do it accurately and fluently (at full speed) and also to generalise it to a range of contexts, e.g., personal self-defence whether an attacker comes from the front, side on or behind.	■	■				
Feedback on behaviour	Present a slide giving feedback on current practice, e.g. results of a recent audit in their hospital or anonymous feedback from a needs assessment, to help bring the issues of the training to life.	■				■	
Prompts and cues	Give learners a resource to prompt the practice and ask them to share where they think it will work best, e.g. putting hand hygiene posters above the sinks in operating theatres.		■	■			■
Problem solving (including Coping planning)	Ask learners in small groups to identify what might get in the way of their new practice in real life and then come up with specific solutions they could use to overcome these.		■	■	■		
Credible source or information about others' approval	Prepare materials featuring stories or case studies from a credible source, talking about their views in favour of the practice, including videos, written narratives and podcasts.				■	■	
Action planning	Ask learners to make a detailed plan about what they will do and when. Link in cues that automatically prompt, using an 'if-then' plan, for example 'if an older person tells me they are struggling with loneliness, I will offer to link them with our social prescribing team'.			■			■
Persuasion about capability	Positively encourage your learners by saying things like 'you are really skilled already; these are just small tweaks', 'we know you can do this' and 'this will become second nature'.		■				
Practical and emotional social support	In small groups, ask participants to articulate how they could gain and give support to each other to help put the new idea into action.		■	■	■		

CAPABILITY

All training courses aim to build learners' knowledge and skills. What makes the best ones stand out? There are many things that are important in creating strong learning memories but one of the most critical is pitching the course at the right level so that it helps to build people's capabilities. Psychological studies tell us that the most effective courses are ones which start from where the learning is needed and upskill the trainees. They build training courses which use 'scaffolding' (providing supportive activities to develop learning, Vygotsky, 1978). This means both you as training leaders and your learners need to know what learners already know (knowledge) and what they already *can* do (skills), either through your scoping work (see Chapter 3) or through training activities. This is, of course, different to what your learners *intend* to do or what they *actually* do in their busy real lives; that's where opportunity and motivation come in.

At the outset of a course, it can be important to highlight, sensitively, as former US Defence Secretary Donald Rumsfeld would put it, your learners' 'known knowns' and 'known unknowns'. Sometimes, learners have a good understanding of what they do and don't know and have chosen your course accordingly, for example signing up to a beginner foreign language class. Many education studies have shown that we are not actually very good at judging our own capability – the most confident learners are not necessarily competent when their skills are tested (Clanton et al. 2014). This can be for many reasons. Individuals sometimes overestimate their competence, particularly in skills that they are using everyday but perhaps have not been using accurately. Nevertheless, they can think that because they are using them, they must have those skills. This is very common in communication skills for example. People will often say 'my friends tell me I'm a great listener' but chatting to friends can be different to the type of listening required in professional practice where the patient or individual needs to actively 'hear' the practitioner listening. In other words, by using reflective listening or active listening, the practitioner *demonstrates* listening. Similarly, people often believe that they are good at setting goals and this may well be true, but these goals may not have the precision that we would expect in a goal-setting exercise. People can also be uncomfortable about revealing what they perceive to be weaknesses around knowledge or skills gaps. For these reasons, training evaluations can frequently show reduced confidence after training; trainers may have done an excellent job of helping learners develop a better understanding of their 'known unknowns'. Nobody is sure who said this, but it might have been Socrates,

Aristotle or the Oracle at Delphi, *'The more I learn, the more I realise how much I don't know.'* As trainers, we need to 'prepare the ground' for learning, developing learners' curiosity and interest to build capability.

What Does the Evidence Say?

Donald Rumsfeld's 'known unknowns' quote maps to the 'Johari Window' (Figure 4), a two-by-two table where what we know/don't know is tabulated against what others know/don't know. In this way, we can identify things that we know we know, things we know we don't know, things we don't realise we know and things we don't realise we don't know (Luft and Ingham 1955).

	Known by self	Unknown by self
Known by others	Things we know we know and are known by others	Things others know but we don't know
Unknown by others	Things we know we know but are hidden to others	Unknown to self and others (things we don't realise we don't know nor do others)

FIGURE 4   The Johari Window.

Tips and examples

Ways of exploring and highlighting capability:

Quizzes and puzzles: Which help learners gauge their own capabilities (privately, never being forced to reveal scores); surprise at unexpected answers can foster engagement.

Example: Learners asked to guess how often patients and their diabetes nurses can correctly recall three goals immediately following consultations; answer is surprisingly low, highlighting need for better communication practices.

Feedback on recent audits: Which might have been done as part of scoping or relate to the need for training. These are best if they're *recent*, *relevant* to the audience and *recommendations* can clearly follow on. Trainers may wish to use 'we' not 'you' language.

Example: In hand hygiene training 'only 31% of people surveyed knew the 5 moments of hand hygiene, so there may be an opportunity for a refresher of our knowledge'.

Case study: Talk through a recent case study asking learners to input what they would ask or do next.

Example: In safeguarding training 'so what would you be asking the family members here at this point, what part of our local guidelines would you look up, who would you need to call for advice?'

Explore meanings: Ask what do we mean by a capable or effective practitioner?

Example: What are the skills and knowledge and practices of an effective practitioner? Ask people to spend some time thinking about how they define being capable or effective in their work. That helps to start from a point of strength and builds a strong sense of community. This is a more general sense of capable and not specific to being 'capable' of the specific IBOs. We often invite people to use pictures and post-it notes to help create an image of an effective practitioner (Figure 5), or they can draw an animal that has the characteristics of an effective practitioner and label the characteristics.

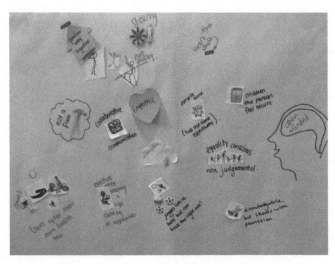

FIGURE 5   Post-it notes to illustrate an effective practitioner.

Building Psychological Capability

There are many ways to develop capability in education and training. We have some top choices, which are partly based on evidence and partly on our own experiences. Educators are often very good at targeting capabilities, because of the focus on competency-based education and assessment in health professional education.

Our top choice BCTs for psychological capability and tips for using them are (see Table 1):

- Instruction on how to perform the behaviour
- Demonstration of the behaviour
- Behavioural practice and rehearsal
- Prompts and cues
- Problem solving
- Persuasion about capability
- Practical and Emotional social support

Tips for using these:

Use (anonymised) stories and step-by-step instructions that bring facts and guidelines to life for your learners.

Practicing and rehearsing rhymes ('C3, 4, 5 – Keeps The Diaphragm Alive!') and mnemonics (5Hs and Ts of cardiac arrest) can be helpful for memorising lists.

Consider whether you can translate guidelines and instructions into different languages – if so, be sure to double check if this is making sense through back translation.

You can build people's confidence (self-efficacy) as you go along, for example with encouragement based on your experience such as 'other people have found this hard to start with but they found that they were able to do this after practicing'. Consider including a (real) story of people, like the group of people you are training, who believed they could not do the IBO but then learned and now are doing it in practice.

Tips and examples

Step-by-step example

What: Case study discussion activity

Time: 20 minutes activity

Aim: To build knowledge about infection control and encourage health-care workers to refer to guidelines

How: Trainer gives out case study to small groups along with relevant guidelines

Example: The healthcare worker (HCW) has only recently started working at the hospital. She has so far received no training but the ward is understaffed and she is asked to attend to patients. There are four patients. She goes from one patient to the next providing them with water and asking them how they feel. The patients are so pleased to see her.

Discuss: What should the HCW do to help protect the patients and herself from infection? What are the risks?
Group then comes back together to discuss learning.

How did it work? *Use of a hypothetical case study can help learners build knowledge, sharing ideas about difficult scenarios whilst feeling safe in a small group setting.*

Building Physical Capability

Our top choice BCTs for building physical capability are (see Table 1):

- Instruction on how to perform the behaviour
- Demonstration of the behaviour
- Behavioural practice and rehearsal
- Feedback on behaviour

Tips for using these:

- When demonstrating, it can be fun and interesting to show the 'wrong way' but make sure you spend more time demonstrating the right way of doing things, so that learners know the behaviour to repeat in their real-life practice. It can be engaging to ask learners to model the behaviour, e.g. reading from a script, rather than the trainer always being the 'expert'.
- Design activities that will develop necessary skills, using practice and rehearsal in graded steps, to help learners first 'acquire' the skill or

skills, then become more fluent and automatic before generalising for use in different settings (Haring, Lovitt, Eaton and Hansen, 1978). When doing demonstration and practice and rehearsal, follow the pattern in Figure 6 (repeat as often as appropriate) which links to Pendelton's rules (Pendelton et al. 1984).

- Feedback (or evaluation below) helps to build capability (as well as motivation) if delivered well. A feedback cycle allows individuals to apply the learning from feedback into the next opportunity to practice the skill.

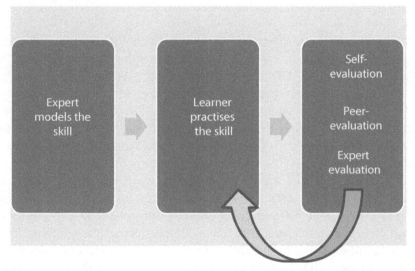

FIGURE 6   A cycle for physical capability improvement (learning a skill).

Tips and examples

What: Learning cardio-pulmonary resuscitation (CPR)

Time: 1 hour session

Aim: To improve healthcare workers' physical capability to perform CPR in a range of situations

How:

1. Trainers demonstrate on a CPR mannequin on a table how to check for signs of life, call for help and start CPR if necessary, beginning by slowly describing each step and then in real time.

2. Participants take turns practising these same steps, first slowly, then more quickly. Each time, they describe the steps they are doing, to reinforce these. Participants, peers and trainers offer feedback after each time.
3. Trainers model steps in different situations, e.g. what if the person is fully clothed, sitting up but unconscious, what if the person is a baby or child?
4. Practice and evaluation continue in a range of situations, until fluency in a range of situations (over rehearsal) is achieved.

Opportunity

Capability and opportunity go hand-in-hand. Capability means we can capitalise on opportunities; taking those opportunities helps maintain and build on our capability. Training is a chance to step back from our busy work life and reflect on what gets in the way of good practice which might not be so obvious to us when we are operating at speed in real-life settings where we may just resort to habit. Opportunity barriers can be identified and openly discussed, with problem-solving skills used to overcome them where possible.

It is important for trainers working with learners from highly pressurised work environments to be sensitive to the many demands on their time and energy. The Karasek Job Demands Control Social Support model (Karasek 1979, Karasek and Theorell 1990) tells us that the combination of high demands and low control and support at work is toxic and predictive of burnout, yet sadly all too familiar to many working in health and social care. Some opportunity problems, such as access to the right resources, may not be immediately 'solvable' but providing a space to reflect on tricky issues can support teams to find ways forward, including safety concerns.

Building Physical Opportunity

Our top choice BCTs for building physical opportunity (see Table 1).

- Prompts and cues
- Problem solving
- Action planning
- Coping planning
- Practical social support

Tips for using these:

- Prompts and cues need to be accessible at the point of performance, e.g. visible laminated posters. Site visits may be needed to co-design suitable prompts.
- Action plans can be in the forms of 'pledges' made at the end of training and should specify exactly what participants plan to do next in their work setting to implement an aspect of training.

Tips and examples

IBO: The nurse (WHO) will do a foot health check (WHAT) with people with type 1 diabetes (TO WHOM) in routine appointments (WHEN, WHERE).

Learning activity: An activity in which learners will increase their perceptions of physical and social opportunity by **defining barriers and** then **problem solving** (particularly time, equipment, other people). Problem solving might include all the ways they could mitigate those barriers by planning, introducing changes to the environment and thinking through how they might handle difficult conversations.

1. Trainer puts a poster on the wall of two people in a consultation and asks people to think of all the things that get in the way of the practitioner asking about, and checking, the patient's foot health. You can ask people to write ideas on the poster or on a separate sheet of paper.
2. Once you have a few ideas, you can even ask two people to demonstrate the problems to others by simulating the situation.
3. Ask the group if they can think of any solutions for these issues. Problem solve together by creating action and coping plans. The more ideas the better, then the group has more to choose from. Coping plans are 'if-then' statements where you specify what you will do if a particular barrier arises. For example, if a group identify that they forget to ask younger people about their foot health because they most often (but not always) have good foot health, they might decide to ask a team secretary to add a reminder to the electronic patient record of all their patients under age 35. Their 'if-then' statement might then be:

'If I am having an appointment with a young person with type 1 diabetes and I forget to ask them about their feet then I will look at the screen reminder when it pops up and remember'.

An Appreciative Inquiry Approach

There is an approach to improvement called 'appreciate inquiry' (Cooperrider 2012). In this approach, instead of focusing on what is hard or challenging we encourage people to focus on what is going well, now and if they were looking back from the future. Theoretically, this is important as we create the narrative of ourselves and our professional roles as we talk about them. If we constantly focus on what is not going well, then our whole story can become one of failure. In the above example, we could ask people to visualise themselves in a year's time where all the change has been made and ask them how they managed it. This subtle change in language means that people are not directed to focus on what they can't do but rather on what their future self-accomplished. Care must be taken not to stifle real implementation issues that learners might be bringing with them. In the approach, it is OK to discuss difficulties, but to be sure to balance with successes (see Further Reading).

Building Social Opportunity

Our top choice BCTs for building social opportunity (see Table 1).

- Information about social consequences
- Problem solving
- Credible source
- Information about others' approval
- Practical and Emotional social support

Tips for using these:

- It can be useful to offer information about positive social consequences (e.g., your service users will thank you for this best practice) rather than only negative consequences.
- Credible sources differ between groups and it's important to explore this in scoping so that the right source is used to build social opportunity. For example, when delivering antimicrobial resistance training to health professionals in Sub-Saharan Africa, doctors had concerns that research underpinning national and international guidelines was not applicable (and so credible) in their context.
- Social support: When individuals will be working together in the practice setting it can be worth exploring how they will support each other

in practicing the new skills. Even if not in the same workplace setting but in the same work roles, people can often get a sense of support from the shared challenges and the shared ambitions to implement new skills. At the end of the course, it can be a good idea to ask people to articulate how they could gain support and give support to each other.

Tips and examples

Developing a menopause-friendly workforce: behaviourally focused e-learning

Aim: An introductory e-learning module aimed to overcome menopause stigma in a large healthcare workforce.

IBO: Workers will discuss menopause (using menopause-friendly language) with their colleagues experiencing menopause during typical workday conversations.

How: To enhance perceptions of social approval and social consequences, an introductory animated video with positive, diverse images and welcoming music highlighted quotes gathered from a range of staff who had attended a scoping focus group. The quotes included those from both individuals directly affected, and their colleagues, on how important this issue is to them (social opportunity). Colleagues experiencing menopause highlighted that using menopause-friendly language and offering personalised support made them feel much more supported at work.

Tips and examples

What: Encouraging people to wear face masks

Time: 1 hour

Aim: To enable those working in volunteer settings to feel competent and confident in asking people to wear face masks.

How:

1. You could start this by asking small groups to use a 3–4 box comic book strip (such as in a small template below) to visually illustrate the

issues around what can happen when volunteers ask members of the public to use face masks.

2. Then ask each group to present their comic book strip and invite the group to consider what each person might be thinking. This helps to move away from entrenched thinking and allows the participants to consider different people's perspectives on the issue.

3. Ask each group to pick up a cartoon strip that they did not create and think of what the options might be for how they could respond (e.g., Figure 7)

4. Discuss as a group.

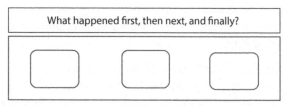

FIGURE 7   Comic book strip. *In the squares show first of all what is the problem. In the next box demonstrate what could be said in response to the situation.*

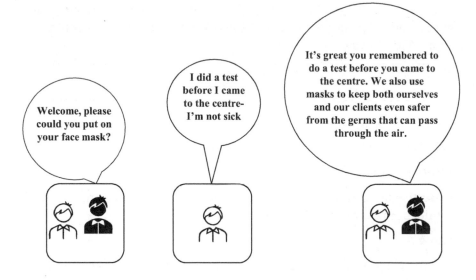

MOTIVATION

Motivation is a wide-ranging concept including our attitudes and things we intend to do but also our automatic habits and routines and emotions. Sometimes in training, we can assume that we will change motivation by persuading that something is a good thing (outcome expectancies), not realising that our audience is already convinced but don't have the habits in routines yet in place. Addressing this through training activities can help learners implement their new skills in action.

BUILDING REFLECTIVE MOTIVATION

Our top choice BCTs for building reflective motivation (see Table 1).

- Goal setting (behaviour)
- Information about health, social or environmental consequences
- Pros and cons
- Feedback on behaviour
- Credible source
- Information about others' approval

Reflective motivation relates to both how inherently good/fun/moral/interesting an idea we think something is (our behavioural attitude), and what we think are the consequences of doing it (our outcome expectancies). Linking to the previous section, we are often more motivated to have a go at a new thing if we feel confident that we can do it. To help build positive **outcome expectancies**, articulate what the better end points are – who will benefit from the IBO and why. Studies show that communication containing both statistics and individual stories can help people understand why something is beneficial and to whom; and that the story should be told, or be about, someone who is credible: often a leader or someone like the learners themselves. Create some stories, slides, handouts, etc. about the positive endpoints of each IBO. You might also consider asking the learners what they think might improve if they do this IBO. If they are not sure, reiterate the outcome benefits. To help build positive **behavioural attitudes** towards doing the new behaviour (all the good things about it), design activities in which learners discuss what it would be like to do the IBO in practice (or what it is like if they have done it before) and ask them to think about whether there is anything they can do to make it easier or more acceptable.

Tips and examples

What: Pros and cons reflections on implications of using motivational interviewing skills in their health promotion practice

Time: 20 minutes

Aim: To help community health workers reflect on the pros and cons of making changes to their practice

How: Ask people to draw a picture of how it would feel or what implications there would be if they were using more skills aligned with a motivational interviewing approach (e.g., open questions, active listening, exploring readiness for change) in their practice, including pros and cons. Then ask individuals to walk about the room and explain their pictures to the rest of the group, starting with any cons raised and moving to pros (also, this picture shows...)

Building Automatic Motivation

Top Choice BCTs for Building Automatic Motivation

- Prompts and cues
- Action planning

Prompts and cues are really powerful drivers of behaviour. Studies suggest that over half of what we do each day is 'automatic' – done on 'autopilot' with little conscious effort, based on our routines (past behaviour). Many of us will help ourselves or family members by setting up reminders, whether a note on the door reminding us to bring our lunch to work, or the more 'natural' prompt of our hungry pet's reminders when it is their breakfast time!

It can be useful to raise awareness of this among busy learners. Ask people to think about their journey to work that day. What can they remember of that journey. For many, it is likely to be very little, because so much of our journeys to work tend to be automatic. We turn left at that street without thinking, we drive the car or walk without having to consciously think about what we are doing. This is a good example of automatic thinking, to show the need for us to plan ways to build new habits.

Making 'if-then' plans can also support automatic motivation but this time instead of coping with something that might get in the way, you can encourage them to use if-then plans to make a plan that cues them if they see a particular cue. For example, if you wanted someone to follow the five-moments of hand hygiene, you might get them to make an if-then plan like: 'If I approach a patient's bed, then I will take the hand gel from my pocket and sanitise my hands'.

Once they have written these, it's worth considering asking people to role play these situations for them to test out how easy it would be, what might get in the way, how they might resolve any of these barriers.

Tips and examples

What: Design your perfect prompting environment

Time: 20 minutes

Aim: To help ward staff remember to ask patients if they have any allergies on admission.

IBO: Ward staff will ask patients if they have any allergies on admission.

How: Be in the ward space or give learners a ward map, either on paper or lego. Ask the learners to design prompts that can help everyone to ensure the IBO is completed. Ideas could be to do with admission paperwork, a poster, or it might be moving where equipment is kept.

PLANNING THE 'HOW' OF YOUR TRAINING

As well as the 'what' we will do in our training, it's wise to plan the basics of 'how' we will do it. Delivering training requires that you think about the environment in which people will learn best.

Consider Space

If the training is to be held in person, space or spaces need to be large enough with enough flexible seating for both larger 'plenary sessions' and smaller breakout group activities. The venue needs to be accessible to all, ideally with easy transport options, so learners can arrive on time and focus on your training, rather than the distraction of how to travel home or avoid a parking fine!

Consider Numbers

How many learners you include in your training may depend on practical issues like scheduling or room availability. For typical behaviourally based training, you may wish to aim for approximately 10–25 learners. This allows enough trainees to generate some good discussions whilst at the same time make it more manageable to ensure you can 'hear' each trainee and monitor and manage the training.

Consider Acoustics and Visuals

Look for spaces that allow the trainer to be seen and heard clearly (considering diversity issues such as visual/auditory impairments among learners, or differences in first language or accent/dialect between trainers and learners which may make learning more difficult), avoiding places with many distractions and interruptions.

Consider Time

As a new trainer, it can be tempting to pack lots of activities into a schedule. Learning needs time for people to reflect on the learning (more of this below) for it to have an impact.

Consider Dynamics

Are you inviting people from the same profession or team, or others, are there hierarchies/dynamics in the team that you need to know about? Perhaps learners might feel more safe to explore and make mistakes if they are not in the same group as their managers, or perhaps managers would help a team implement change together? This is one to explore in advance when you have the luxury of having this option. Frequently, you will not be able to choose. Discussing this at the very outset of a course as part of the ground rules can help build people's comfort with group leaders.

Consider Technical Equipment and Skills

Make plans (and back-up plans!) to ensure presentations and activities can run effectively, whether training is in person or online.

Consider Administrative Support

For advertising, booking, printing of any materials and smooth running.

Consider Refreshments

These can seem trivial and be overlooked where budgets are limited but make learners feel valued members of a learning partnership and help ensure people can focus on training, particularly in hospitals or low resource settings. When we have done training in low-resource settings, learners have often come straight from a night shift to attend training and are in much need of food and caffeine. This is all part of creating a nurturing and collaborative training environment!

Consider Culture/Contexts/Countries

It's good practice to be sensitive to the cultures, contexts and countries in which you are delivering training. Parachuting into a training situation without taking local cultures, beliefs and practices into account can mean at best, the training will be meaningless and of little value. At worst, it can lead to people taking offence. To avoid that, be certain to collaborate with the local training commissioners at the outset. Check your assumptions and understanding of what is required. What are normal practices and procedures and any particular considerations that you should be taking into account? Building the training collaboratively with the commissioners and key stakeholders gives a much greater likelihood that the training will be appropriate for the context and culture. It is as important to think about local cultures and practices in other countries as it is to apply it to a particular setting within the country in which you are resident. In different settings, people frequently have particular ways of doing things, ways of perceiving things which can vary from setting to setting. Becoming familiar with these, and providing space for them, will increase the likelihood of the effectiveness of the training. In most settings, taking account of dietary needs of participants is important and helps them feel valued. In some cultures and settings it is the norm for learners to have a space and time for prayer during the day, for example. Issues of religion and culture may need to be openly, sensitively discussed and planned for if e.g., mixed gender volunteer training in certain islamic countries. In some cultures and settings, learners usually receive a 'per diem' or payment to attend continuing professional development, and this too frequently applies to the training of volunteers. Trainers need to discuss such cultural considerations in advance with those commissioning the training learners/managers.

ONLINE

Increasingly, training is delivered through a combination of some face-to-face (f2f) elements and some online elements referred to as a hybrid or blended learning approach. In a blended learning approach it is even more important that participants know what to expect, when to expect it, and have the skills to engage with whatever medium your teaching will be delivered through.

Teaching online means that you may need to spend some time providing guidance about how to access the learning, which will depend on the functionality of the platform. This may mean guiding people how to access a Zoom© or TEAMS© meeting by providing pre-training notes, specifically around how to access. You may also need to consider thinking through different guidelines about how people interact. Do you want people to speak whenever they choose, or would you prefer for people to use the 'raise the hand' function? And you will also need to consider whether you want people to keep their cameras on or off. Keeping cameras on can be very helpful to build a sense of community in your training. But there may be issues if your participants are working from home and there are children nearby, or if they are sharing a space with others in the room. These may be barriers to being able to fully participate or engage in the training. It may be useful for a co-facilitator to monitor the chat function. Many of us will have experienced the whirl of activity in online meetings and you will want to be 'fully present' for your participants. If it is a large group, how will you use breakout rooms? We'd suggest, from hard-won experience, being clear about what time and how to return to the main group to be very important to avoid people waiting around or lost in cyberspace. It is useful to let people know if you will be 'popping in' to the breakout groups to offer help and advice, to avoid giving participants a big surprise!

BLENDED LEARNING – SYNCHRONOUS AND ASYNCHRONOUS

We use the term 'synchronous' to describe learning which is taking place at the same time, for example a webinar happening in real time on a conferencing platform like Zoom. Asynchronous learning can take place at different times and includes videos that have been pre-recorded, quizzes and discussion boards.

How you manage the different components is up to you, but there is a lot of benefit in providing some information before the participants and you meet, followed by some synchronous learning and perhaps asynchronous learning through discussion board or personal reflections interspersed during that time. It will also depend on the length of the course and what you are trying to achieve.

Pre-course information might consist of a document outlining information about how to access the course, objectives of the course and perhaps even some of the ground rules (which you can discuss further and check for agreement to these at the first session). This could be accompanied by a video of you telling them about what to expect and how the course will operate; this can help to make it more personal. Pre-course information is also an opportunity to provide some questions you want people to think about or tasks you want people to do in advance of the course, for example, having the information to allow them to test the learning platform, questions that help them to consider aspects that will be discussed on the course (*what gets in the way of using handgel when you are seeing patients*), or perhaps watching a little video of people using or not using handgel in a clinic environment. The online synchronous training should be tasks that are best done together and which are more interactive, and then or example where discussion is useful, where there is a demonstration, or when you want to be certain what people have understood from the training. During these synchronous sessions, as you would do in a face-to-face learning environment, you can also pause for a bit of time, providing participants with Power-Points, a website to look at or some reading and/or an activity, then invite the participants to come back to the online platform to discuss. In online learning, do remember to give many breaks. Intensive screen time can be demanding and very tiring.

What students learn online can be equivalent to what they learn face to face (Maltinsky et al. 2013), but it does require careful planning so that participants not only feel engaged with the delivery of the learning but have no problems accessing the digital technology. In other words, they need the digital literacy skills required. Some factors are important for online learning (see Further Reading, particularly Hung et al. 2010). Figure 8 summarises considerations when preparing a blended learning programme.

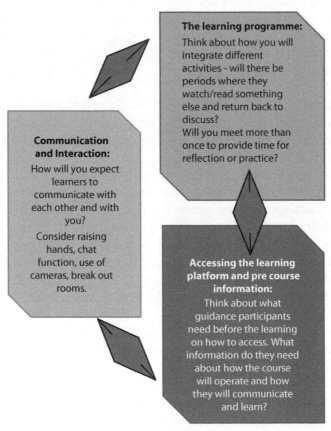

FIGURE 8   Considerations for a blending learning course.

THE BUILDING BLOCKS OF YOUR TRAINING

Regardless of the number of days and of the platform you use for training, a typical behaviourally informed training may look similar to that in Figure 9.

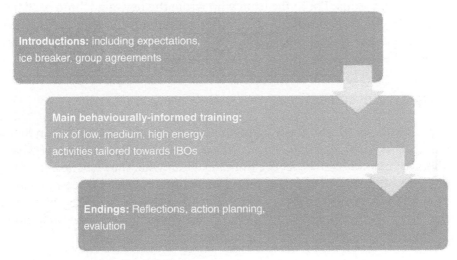

Introductions: including expectations, ice breaker, group agreements

Main behaviourally-informed training: mix of low, medium, high energy activities tailored towards IBOs

Endings: Reflections, action planning, evalution

FIGURE 9   Overview of training structure.

Beyond this, it can be useful to make a more detailed training plan using a form like the examples for two different kinds of training given in the Guides (examples 1 and 2), linked back to BCTs.

INTRODUCTIONS

Welcoming

Make certain that individuals are welcomed into the training space and that it is set out ready for the training. It can be daunting to walk into a training environment, so do what you can to make people feel welcome. If possible, offer refreshments, but at the very least, welcome and introduce yourselves and direct them to where they can sit.

Introductory Activities

People in a course can often struggle with being the first person to speak out loud, therefore this task needs to fall to you as the trainer. Spend a few minutes introducing yourself which can also include your credibility as a trainer: 'I'm X and I'm a consultant haematologist with 20 years of experience in Sickle Cell anaemia, I'm in the team who wrote the new guidelines we'll be talking about today'. Introduce the course and present the objectives of the training, demonstrating your openness and flexibility to listening to the needs of the trainees.

Trainee Introductions

Everyone sits waiting for the rounds of introductions anticipating when they will be required to speak. For some, this may mean they hear little of what others have said because they are thinking about what they will need to say. Make it a bit easier for people by using some different techniques and making it a bit more fun. The following ice breaker activities can take a bit more time but can be valuable for making people feel more comfortable and building that collaborative training environment:

Create Name-Plates

You can receive strange looks when people first walk into the room and spot the colouring pens, paper, scissors and prompt words and pictures but then people get engrossed in the task of creating a name-plate, sitting at a table with others and during that time they also start to chat to their neighbours. The initial sense of anxiety of starting a new course starts to dissipate. You can give people some helpful pictures that they can glue to their page (cut-out from magazines or printed icons) which makes it easier for those who feel they 'have no talent'. A name-plate could be a favourite pastime, job role, a surprise that others don't know about them, and you can even ask them to jot down a hope for the course. These can be pinned to the wall or if you are sitting at desks, placed on the desk. You can ask each person to introduce themselves or a partner who they have chatted to for a few minutes before the introductions.

Introductory Bingo

Write a list of things to collect on a grid and hand out to each trainee. Their task is to find a different person for each item on their list. For example, 'Find someone who... is wearing red socks, who likes (a particular food), who can roll their tongue into a curve, who has been on night shift....' You can adapt this list to whatever group you are working with. At the end of the bingo game, you can ask questions such as, 'Did you find out something about someone you didn't know before? What was a surprise; what did you know before?'

Introduce Your Neighbour

Ask people to talk to their neighbour and find out what they do, what they like and one thing about this person you didn't know before or one thing they were thinking as they were coming into the training today (keeping it to three questions will make it easier to remember). Then ask people to introduce their neighbours.

Throw the Soft Toy

A fast and easy game (and which can be repeated throughout the course) is to throw a soft toy (you can also roll a ball, or pass the item depending on abilities in the group) and ask only one question at a time, for example, 'name one thing you were thinking as you travelled to the training, one thing you noticed on your journey.'

GROUP AGREEMENTS

There are arguments for and against introducing group agreements before the introductions or after. It can be really useful for you to do so at the outset because it then covers anything that might be said in the introductions. Group agreements can feel more formal and so without the lightness of the individual introductions, not everyone might be as comfortable to contribute. One option is to make your agreements at the outset and then return to it after the introductions and ask people if they want to add or adapt anything.

You can list out some common headings in the group agreements such as confidentiality, listening to all voices, phones switched off or to silent, respect for each other. Allow people time to speak to these and to add or adapt any that are appropriate. This can be done as a whole group exercise or ask people to talk in twos or threes and report back.

Course Expectations, Hopes and Fears

It's a very good idea to get an understanding of how people are feeling about the course and what they hope to get out of it. This can also be tied into the group agreements. Many, for example, will be fearful of having to speak out in front of a group, knowing from the group agreement that this is not required and that you as the trainer will facilitate group discussions that allow their voices to be heard without having to speak up, can be comforting. For this activity, it can be useful to post three different sheets on the wall and ask people to go to these sheets and write up their expectations, hopes and fears.

Balancing Training Energy

Your training should also consider how to manage energy levels. Include some 'higher energy', fun or movement-based activities as well as some lower-energy, more reflective activities. Avoid at all costs the risks of death by PowerPoint. If using PowerPoint, always follow this up with an activity that allows people to demonstrate their understanding of that concept. Low-energy tasks are frequently PowerPoint demonstrations, paired or small group talking but can be some moments in which individuals reflect individually. Moderate energy tasks can be in groups writing thoughts/ideas on large sheets of paper (graffiti charts) and also walking around the room looking at other groups' charts. Higher-energy tasks are those that are active and use some energy. These can be role plays or more advanced forms of role plays, such as having the main 'characters' swapping seats with others in the 'audience' every two minutes. Some fun activities such as 'building' using creative activities are also high energy. Building the setting can be fun and can get people into the spirit of thinking about the workplace, its setting, how it's used, who uses it and what are normal practices that occur in those spaces. This is where we collect our post, the cakes donated by visitors are always piled onto this table. You can make this 'building' expansive or simple. It will depend on your resources the space and the time available as well as your objectives. Building the space can be about setting up the training room to mimic the workspace using pictures or other objects to symbolise objects from the workspace, e.g. 'we'll use this chair to represent the sink'. The advantage of setting up the room in this way is that it allows you to talk about things that might be habitual by members but they hadn't realised. It's also now available for you to use to practice some role plays. Alternatively, you can use large sheets of paper in which groups draw the space. Again, making this a large activity brings more energy with it, with several people working on the same sheet or small sheets of paper where individuals create their own view of the workspace and then compare.

ENDINGS: REFLECTION, ACTION PLANNING AND EVALUATION

If not included as an explicit learning activity, it can be useful to build in plenty of time at the end of the training session for reflection about new learning and thoughts about how participants will put in practice the knowledge, skills and confidence they've acquired during training. Your learners may also feel a shared sense of identity and support which you could foster using a champion network and sharing of contact details.

We cover evaluation in Chapter 5, but it is worth thinking about how education and training activities can form part of evaluation too. The activities that require people to plan for change can be recorded in some way and then analysed to see if learners have experienced the training in the way intended. For example, if you have included a session around overcoming barriers and solutions to changing practice but learners in the action planning session are still wondering about the same barriers, it is reasonable to conclude that the earlier session might need revising.

CHECK YOUR UNDERSTANDING AND REFLECT

1. Which aspects and activities/resources used in education and training are likely to contain Behaviour Change Techniques (BCTs)?
2. How do we move from gathering influences on behaviour to choosing BCTs?
3. Give an example of a BCT used in CPD which targets a) capability, b) opportunity and c) motivation.
4. How can an appreciative inquiry approach be helpful in CPD courses?

5. If you were to ask learners to get into pairs and weigh up their personal positives and down sides of making a certain change to their practice, which BCT would this be?
6. What is the value of including a mix of low-, medium- and high-energy training activities in CPD?
7. Thinking back to an education/training session you've taken part in as a learner, how did the nine practical considerations (e.g., space, numbers, administration) feel from your perspective? Would you organise any of these differently if you had been the course leader?

FURTHER READING

For more appreciate inquiry see https://www.davidcooperrider.com/ai-process.

For an overview of feedback in clinical settings see Burgess, A., van Diggele, C., Roberts, C., and Mellis, C. (2020). Feedback in the clinical setting. *BMC Medical Education* 20 (460). https://doi.org/10.1186/s12909-020–02280-5.

To learn more about how behaviour change techniques are linked to theories and mechanisms of action see https://theoryandtechniquetool.human behaviourchange.org/tool.

For blended/online learning

https://www.gillysalmon.com/five-stage-model.html

https://www.benjanefitness.com/blendedlearning

Hung, M.L., Chou, C., Chen, C.H., and Own, Z.Y. (2010). Learner readiness for online learning: Scale development and student perceptions. *Computers & Education* 55 (3): 1080–1090.

REFERENCES

Bull, E.R. and Dale, H. (2021). Improving community health and social care practitioners' confidence, perceived confidence and intention to use behaviour change techniques in health behaviour change conversations. *Health and Social Care in the Community* 29: 280–283.

Byrne-Davis, L.M.T., Bull, E.R., and Hart, J.K. (2022) Co-creating behaviour change technique activities with people who will deliver them: the Cards for Change.Annals of Behavioural Medicine (in press).

Clanton, J., Gardner, A., Cheung, M., Mellert, L., Evancho-Chapman, M., and George, R.L. (2014). The relationship between confidence and competence in the development of surgical skills. *Journal of Surgical Education* 71 (3): 405–412.

Cooperrider, D. (2012) Appreciative inquiry. https://www.davidcooperrider. com/ai-process (accessed 4 July 2022).

Haring, N.G., Lovitt, T.C., Eaton, M.D., & Hansen, C.L. (1978). The fourth R: Research in the classroom. Columbus, OH: Charles E. Merrill Publishing Co.Karasek, R.A. (1979). Job demands, job decision latitude, and mental strain: implications for job redesign. *Administrative Science Quarterly* 24: 285–308.

Karasek, R.A. and Theorell, T. (1990). *Healthy Work*. New York: Basic Books.

Luft, J. and Ingham, H. (1955). The Johari window, a graphic model of interpersonal awareness. In: *Proceedings of the Western Training Laboratory in Group Development*. Los Angeles: University of California, Los Angeles.

Maltinsky, W., Hall, S., Grant, L., Simpson, K., and MacRury, S. (2013). Pilot project and evaluation of delivering diabetes work-based education using video conferencing. *Rural and Remote Health* 13 (1): 2053.

Michie, S., Atkins, L., & West, R. (2014). The behaviour change wheel. *A guide to designing interventions. 1st ed. Great Britain: Silverback Publishing*, 1003–1010.

Michie, S., Richardson, M., Johnston, M., Abraham, C., Francis, J., Hardeman, W., ... & Wood, C. E. (2013). The behavior change technique taxonomy (v1) of 93 hierarchically clustered techniques: building an international consensus for the reporting of behavior change interventions. *Annals of behavioral medicine*, 46(1), 81–95.

Pearson, E., Byrne-Davis, L., Bull, E., & Hart, J. (2020). Behavior change techniques in health professional training: developing a coding tool. *Translational Behavioral Medicine*, 10(1), 96–102.

Pendelton, D., Schofield, T., Tate, P., and Havelock, P. (1984). *The Consultation: An Approach to Learning and Teaching*. Oxford: Oxford University Press.

Vygotsky, L.S. (1978). *Mind in society: The development of higher psychological processes*. Cambridge, MA: Harvard University Press.

CHAPTER 5

Assessing and Evaluating

Learning Points

- Our evaluations should be both of outcomes of training and the process of training, based on our theory of change
- Evaluations can use quantitative and qualitative methods
- Evaluations are most useful when they are used as part of a cycle of quality improvement of your education and training
- Evaluations are best if they compare before and after the training
- Evaluations can be embedded within the training itself to reduce the burden on trainees

Why evaluate? Many years ago, as new trainers, we didn't quite understand the value or importance of evaluating. Surely, if people liked the course, they'd tell us or show us? But then one day, slightly longer in the tooth, we

Training to Change Practice: Behavioural Science to Develop Effective Health Professional Education, First Edition. Jo Hart, Lucie Byrne-Davis, Wendy Maltinsky, and Eleanor Bull. © 2023 John Wiley & Sons Ltd. Published 2023 by John Wiley & Sons Ltd.

came across someone who had participated in one of our training courses. She enthused about the course, the interesting methods we had used and how she felt that her voice was valued and heard. We smiled and glowed, warmed by this confirmation we thought we were hearing about the value of the programme. 'So, how did the course change what you were doing in your setting?', we asked. 'Oh, I didn't change at all. None of it was new, nor did I really think the things that were being taught were that important to use, but I did really like the training and I did feel valued'.

Why we evaluate really helps us consider: why do we train? Most often we train to introduce a new skill or way of doing something or because we want to improve outcomes for our patients or organisations. When we provide knowledge, it is more than often because we are attempting to introduce this knowledge to help people change. Evaluation, therefore, needs to ascertain, not only that people liked the training and learnt new information, but that the objective of the training: to change an element of practice in a setting, has been achieved.

We evaluate to understand more about how our training may be assisting people to implement the new skills/knowledge. We want to know if our training has been effective in helping people to make practice changes. From the story above, hopefully you'll see just how important it is to not simply ask people about how satisfied they are with the training as this does not indicate if they have put the new skills/knowledge into practice. Satisfaction with and acceptability of training is clearly very important but not sufficient for change in practice. Whilst it is not always easy to evaluate whether people are using the new knowledge and skills in the workplace, the rest of this chapter will provide some ideas about how to do so.

PROCESS VS. OUTCOME

The biggest distinction in evaluation is between evaluating the process and evaluating the outcome. Outcome evaluation asks whether your education and training was effective, i.e. did it change what you wanted it to change. Outcomes from education and training are often related to patient morbidity or mortality, but there might be other outcomes such as staff retention or change in resource use. For example, if training is aiming to reduce the use of using letters for communication between consultants in preference to electronic forms to speed up communication channels, then your expectation would be a reduction in letters and postage. By the same token, if you were training on the use of hand gel you would expect more hand gel to be used as one of the outcomes. In research, the specification of outcome is taken very seriously and often there is a distinction made between the primary outcome and any secondary outcomes. For example, you might seek to reduce the number of prescriptions of broad-spectrum antibiotics in a particular patient group or hospital and this is the primary or most important outcome. You might also be interested in patient satisfaction or experience with having or not having an antibiotic prescription, so this might be a secondary outcome.

Process evaluation is also very important. This relates to the theory of change you have developed, and which was discussed in Chapter 2. In your theory of change, you have specified *how* you think your education and training is going to lead to better outcomes. To know whether your education and training is doing what you think it is doing, you can test the theory of change by measuring the steps along the way. For example, did the people we expect to attend actually attend; were the appropriate training resources available for use; did capability, opportunity and motivation about particular behaviours change? The reasons that this is so important are manifold. Firstly, if the education and training does not change the outcome, you will really want to understand why so that you can address this in future deliveries. Secondly, if the outcome is improved, you will want to know how, so that you can learn from that for future projects. Process evaluation can be very useful for quality improvement of education and training if you are to deliver the same training multiple times.

WHY ARE YOU EVALUATING?

The most important thing to decide about evaluation is the reason you are evaluating. If you agree this, as a team, then the decisions about what and how to evaluate will flow from that. Some of the reasons for evaluation will include wanting to know if something has worked to convince a policy maker or funder to invest in your course. Sometimes the reasons are more localised than that. You may want to capture the impact of your course on the people or organisations involved, which also allows you to think about how this training may be of value or need to be adapted for delivery to other similar organisations. Sometimes, evaluation data can be used for research publications, usually if there are some generalisable findings.

THEORIES AND FRAMEWORKS TO HELP US EVALUATE

Evaluation overlaps with research, although evaluation is about the specific education and training (think 'local problem, local solution') whilst research is about generalisable findings. This overlap, however, provides excellent methods to help us think about our evaluations, since often the data collection will be similar. We will introduce some of these methods here, but only briefly, since they have been written about in much more detail elsewhere.

THE KIRKPATRICK MODEL

Perhaps the most well-known structure of evaluation is the Kirkpatrick model (Kirkpatrick 1959), which proposes that there are four 'levels' of evaluation of training. Firstly, level one is how much people like the training, including how relevant they think it is and how engaging they felt it was. This is important for many reasons but perhaps particularly for courses that will take place multiple times, as you want learners to attend and that will be supported if others have said that they liked it and thought it was relevant. Level two assesses learning. This is a common way of evaluating education and training. This will include whether the learners' knowledge or skills have changed, i.e. whether they know, know how and can show how to do something new. It is important to remember that because someone *can* do something doesn't mean that their behaviour will change in a practice setting, so measuring skills is still a level two evaluation. Other features that we have discussed throughout the book, like opportunity and motivation, also are part of level 2. In other words, level two includes many of the behavioural influences we introduced in Chapter 1. Assessing motivation for example may include establishing whether the trainees' plans and/or confidence to implement the new behaviour has increased following the training. Level three is behaviour, and of course directing education and training towards changing behaviour is the purpose of this book. Finally, level four is about outcomes, as we have previously mentioned in this chapter. Understanding the levels of evaluation is very helpful in planning what and why to evaluate.

Tips and examples

Evolved from Kirkpatrick, 1959

Level 1 evaluation: Did you enjoy the training? Was the venue suitable? Was the trainer approachable?

Level 2 evaluation: This is where you evaluate capability, opportunity and motivation for each behaviour.

Level 3 evaluation: This is where you evaluate by behaviour change – do people do the behaviours more often when they get back into work?

Level 4 evaluation: Is there an improvement in outcomes for anyone? For example, are patients better? Is quality of life better? Are staff more engaged/less burnt out? Are there more patients receiving safe care?

EVALUATION OF COMPLEX INTERVENTIONS

The Medical Research Council in the UK have been publishing guidance on how to evaluate complex interventions for many years. A complex intervention is one that targets several behaviours and has multiple, interacting components (Skivington et al. 2021) and education and training is sometimes such an intervention, particularly when it forms part of a wider project. The Medical Research Council guidance states that selection of important measures of outcome, and then assessing at multiple time points, is crucial for good evaluation. Since, as we have explored throughout this book, we are often interested in practice change, we might then seek to measure practice at time points before and after our education and training. Such assessment can be done objectively and subjectively.

Objective measurement could include analysis of routinely collected data, particularly if the education and training was in a specific place of work. For example, if your education and training is about appropriate use of antibiotics, you might audit antibiotic use by conducting a point prevalence survey or you might count the number of a particular type of antibiotic prescriptions. You could also observe people at work using a behavioural checklist. For example, you might be trying to improve patient safety measures, like safe surgical checklists, in the operating room so you might then observe whether these were carried out in line with best practice. Objective measurement is sometimes not possible. Sometimes, the education and training might be delivered to people who have come from a wide range of organisations or you might not have the resources to directly measure outcomes. In these cases, asking people to self-report their behaviours can be an alternative.

Self-report of behaviour is exactly that, you ask people direct questions about how many times they have done a particular behaviour. For example, in the first example of antibiotic prescription, you can ask people to record how many times they have prescribed a particular antibiotic in the last relevant period of time. An appropriate time frame is important because you need there to be enough time that they will have done the behaviour but not too much time so that they can't possibly remember approximate numbers. If asking for these sorts of self-reports, it can also be useful to ask how many patients they saw with whom they *could have* done that behaviour and then with how many they *did* that behaviour. This will help people to delve into their memories and will also give a clearer picture of their behaviour, since for each person you can compare how many they could have done with how many they did.

Process evaluations are so important in complex interventions that they also have their own Medical Research Council guidance (Moore et al. 2015). This guidance provides a really useful framework for process evaluations, including three core components: implementation, mechanisms of change and contextual factors. These link to the theory of change described earlier in the book. You can evaluate process qualitatively, for example with interviews and focus groups, or quantitatively, with questionnaires or direct observations or other numerical data e.g., audit data.

ASSESSING BEHAVIOURAL INFLUENCES

You can assess behavioural influences in two main ways: using questionnaires and by interviews or focus groups. Questionnaires are often used to assess an individual's perceptions. It is easy to see, therefore, how they could be used to assess an individual's perceptions of their knowledge, motivation, capability and so on. It is important, though, that the questions are phrased correctly and that they capture the right aspects of these quite complex constructs. You'll also need to think about whether you're using these just to explore influences and shape your training, or to evaluate your training. If the latter, you'll likely want to ask your group to complete this soon-before and soon-after training, so that you can increase your confidence that any differences in perceptions are due to your training, rather than anything else going on (see this chapter). You will have heard people talk about the validity and reliability of questionnaires. A full discussion of these features is beyond our text, but there are some useful books referenced at the end of this chapter. Unless you have an expert in questionnaires or behavioural science working with you, it is probably safest to stick with some questionnaires that have been used in previous work and for which some tests of validity and reliability have been conducted. There is a direct measure of capability, opportunity and motivation, which has been tested with health professionals (Keyworth et al. 2020). There is a more in-depth, longer questionnaire, that assesses more detailed influences on people's behaviours, called the Theoretical Domains Framework (Huijg et al. 2014). With both of these, you ask each question relating to each intended behavioural outcome you are assessing. You can see how the number of questions might quickly multiply if you have multiple behaviours of interest! In these cases, you can choose to include some example behaviours. You can also decide to assess behaviours one after another, if you hold multiple training courses. For courses that run over again, we have ourselves honed down on one behaviour, measured behavioural influences and then when we know about that behaviour, moved on to assessing the next and so on. Interviews and focus groups are another way to assess behavioural influences. Just as you might have used these to establish the influences that needed to be targeted in the education and training, you can use these to establish the situation in respect of these influences after the education and training. Often, people want to get numbers or 'hard data' but the perceptions of learners about how the influences on behaviours have changed as a result of the education and training can be just as useful. Further, interviews and focus groups might give more insight into why influences might not be changing, in the case where you are not finding much change after your training intervention. For an example of topic guide using the Theoretical Domains Framework, see the box below.

The topic guide in Figure 10 was used in interviews led by psychologists and medical fellows evaluating the World Federation of the Societies of Anaesthesiologist's SAFE Obstetrics training in Tanzania, Nepal and Bangladesh (Dharni et al. in press). They interviewed medical and nursing staff 3 months after training to gain insights into how training had been implemented in practice, including barriers and facilitators, as well as training acceptability.

Topic guide (approx. 45–60 minutes)

On the course
1. Why did you attend the SAFE course in **[LOCATION OF SAFE COURSE]** in **[MONTH]**?
2. What were your expectations of the course?
3. How were your expectations similar or different from reality once you were on the course?
4. If you were to tell a friend about what the SAFE course was about, what would you say?

Since the course
5. What has been the impact of the course for you personally? *Prompts on your confidence, feelings, for you as a nurse/doctor?*
6. How about the impact for mothers and babies?
7. What has been the impact for your team and hospital? *Prompts: What about how you work with your colleagues?*

FIGURE 10   Topic guide example for interviews about the impact of a course on practice at follow-up.

8. Since the course, have you made or noticed any changes in your hospital? *Prompt: What were the changes?*
9. How successfully have these been implemented?
10. What were the challenges/problems?
11. How could these be overcome?
12. What was the reaction of your colleagues and seniors?
13. Can you give us an example of a mother or baby you remember who you managed differently after the course compared to how you used to manage them before the SAFE course?

Prompts: Tell us what you did, when, how, with whom...What was the outcome? Ask – Is there a specific emergency you managed differently? Try to elicit information about several in and out of theatre situations, e.g. before, during and after an operation with a mother?

14. What learning has been difficult to put into practice after you came back from the course? *Prompts: Can you give an example? What have been the issues? Anything else? Try to elicit as much information as possible on this important topic.*
15. What would help overcome these? *Prompt: How could this help?*
16. *Have you been able to use any of the resources you took home from the course? Prompt: Which ones? In what way?*
17. How do you plan to use the learning from the course from now on?

Feedback about the course
18. Overall, what did you think about the safe course? *Prompt: Be sure to ask both – What was good? What was not so good or could be improved for next time?*
19. What aspects of SAFE were new learning for you?
20. And what did you already know before attending SAFE?
21. Now I would like to ask you about the different activities covered in the course. What did you think of ...
    (a) The lectures
    (b) The scenarios
    (c) The skill stations
    (d) The discussion groups
    (e) The materials to take home *Prompt: What could be improved for each?*
22. Thinking of the trainers, what did they do that was good?
23. What could be better next time?

Wrap up and end
24. Is there anything else you would like to say about the SAFE course?

FIGURE 10   (Continued)

25. If there was one message you wanted to tell the people who organised the SAFE obstetrics course, what would it be?

Note: 'Since the course' is the most important section and should be prioritised if time is very short.

FIGURE 10   (Continued)

ASSESSING BEHAVIOUR

As well, or instead of asking people about their thoughts and feelings or to remember behaviours, behaviour can be assessed objectively, through audit, observation or through analysis of routinely collected data. Thousands of audits are registered and conducted in hospitals each year, with the help of diligent, hard-working quality improvement teams for example, on practice behaviours from prescriptions of antibiotics, how often allergies are recorded on drug charts, to surgeries completed without errors. Routinely collected data which could be reanalysed for training evaluation are often related to service targets, for example, numbers of people referred to smoking services in a given timeframe. Observations are often useful where skills needing to be assessed are more subtle, 'soft skills', often not specifically documented or the context is sensitive and would need a skilled approach or permissions. This could be for example, multi-disciplinary team communication in a team with a high level of burn out, or skills used by sexual health advisers when giving contraception advice after an abortion.

These approaches all provide an opportunity for evaluation of training by comparing participants' practices in a period before the training and a time after the training. If your education and training is within one organisation, it is sometimes possible to put together different forms of evaluation data and share findings with audit or quality improvement departments, to add value and insights for teams and departments and highlight your training course as an area of good practice.

It's important to think carefully about who in a training team or organisation might be best to observe teams at work and how to set this up collaboratively. It is important that team members don't feel judged or scrutinised, so usually it would be useful to choose a person who is separate to their management structure and carefully explain to team leaders, teams and (where needed) patients or service users that the purpose is to help understand how easy the course has been to put into practice, to help judge the course, not the learners! The observer needs to have the skills to be warm and friendly and 'blend in', observing practice taking field notes or using observation tools unobtrusively, without correcting team members (unless harm would be caused by not doing so).

Behaviours (as activities people do or don't do) can be recorded on observation tools such as checklists. We would usually include some details around whether the behaviour was expected (i.e., would the training course advocate that this be performed in this context) and then whether it was done at all (i.e., attempted), done to the standard taught on the course, or nearly done, which we sometimes call a 'near miss'. You can see an example of an observation checklist in the 'Guides' section of the book.

CHECK YOUR UNDERSTANDING

1. What is the difference between process and outcome evaluation CPD courses? Can you think of some examples of each?
2. Why is it useful to think about evaluation at each of Kirkpatrick's levels?
3. Which levels and methods are most often used for evaluation in your setting and what are the advantages and disadvantages of the methods used?
4. Imagine you want to evaluate whether a new training changes learners' COM perceptions through a questionnaire. Why would it be important to collect questionnaire data from learners both before and after the course, rather than just asking people directly whether their COM perceptions have changed?
5. Thinking of your next training, how might you bring more behavioural science into its evaluation?

FURTHER READING

https://www.matter-of-focus.com/an-overview-of-the-matter-of-focus-approach

https://evaluationsupportscotland.org.uk/evaluation/evaluation-pathway/
    setting-outcomes-indicators

https://www.gov.uk/guidance/evaluation-in-health-and-wellbeing-outcome

https://evaluationframework.sportengland.org/media/1305/logic-model-
    template.pdf

REFERENCES

Dharni, N., Byrne-Davis, L., Sanga, E., Hart, J., Shrestha, A., Gurung, T., Shrestha, R., Vaidya, P., Hossain, A., Lilaonitkul, M., Snell, D., Barrett-Chapman, A., Walker, I., and Bull, E. (in press) Using Behavioural Science to Explore Impact and Implementation of Obstetric Anaesthesia Training in Tanzania. Nepal and Bangladesh: A qualitative evaluation study with obstetric anaesthesia providers. *Psychology and Health.*

Huijg, J.M., Gebhardt, W.A., Crone, M.R. et al. (2014). Discriminant content validity of a theoretical domains framework questionnaire for use in implementation research. *Implementation Science* 9, 33.

Keyworth, C., Epton, T., Goldthorpe, J., Calam, R., and Armitage, C.J. (2020 September). Acceptability, reliability, and validity of a brief measure of capabilities, opportunities, and motivations ("COM-B"). *British Journal of Health Psychology* 25 (3): 474–501.

Kirkpatrick, D.L. (1959). Techniques for evaluation training programs. *Journal of the American Society of Training Directors* 13: 21–26.

Moore, G.F., Audrey, S., Barker, M., Bond, L., Bonell, C., Hardeman, W. et al. (2015). Process evaluation of complex interventions: medical research council guidance. *BMJ* 350: h1258.

Skivington, K., Matthews, L., Simpson, S.A., Craig, P., Baird, J., Blazeby, J.M., Boyd, K.A., Craig, N., French, D.P., McIntosh, E., Petticrew, M., Rycroft-Malone, J., White, M., and Moore, L. (2021). Framework for the development and evaluation of complex interventions: gap analysis, workshop and consultation-informed update. *Health Technology Assessment* 25 (57).

Guides

SAMPLE TRAINING PLANS

We've included sample training plans annotated to show why the training is planned in this way, according to what you've learnt in this book. These will be most useful if you use them as a guide rather than as a template. We have tried to show the balance of activities as well as how to progress through the day incorporating the relevant BCTs from Capability, Motivation and Opportunity. We commence from the point of assessing knowledge and skills, identifying and building motivation, establishing barriers and facilitators to change, problem solving those changes and finally working towards setting individual plans for change.

Example 1 A brief introduction to hand washing (3-hour session).

TABLE 2 Setting up the session.

Session content	Reasons for inclusion
Intended Behavioural Outcomes (IBOs) After attending the session participants will: Wash their hands each time before they see a patient Wash their hands each time after they complete seeing a patient When a visitor arrives to the clinic, they will ask them to wash their hands before they proceed When they go into the room, they will check to see if they have hand gel	Including IBOs at the start of the session so that learners and tutors are in agreement about the purposes of the session and what learners should be aiming to do differently after the session

(Continued)

Training to Change Practice: Behavioural Science to Develop Effective Health Professional Education, First Edition. Jo Hart, Lucie Byrne-Davis, Wendy Maltinsky, and Eleanor Bull.
© 2023 John Wiley & Sons Ltd. Published 2023 by John Wiley & Sons Ltd.

TABLE 2   *(Continued)*

Session content	Reasons for inclusion
Pre-course material A video clip showing how to hand wash distributed before the session	Using time before sessions for learners to access information about what and how to do simple skills means that more of the contact time can be spent developing complex skills and focusing on developing opportunity and motivation
Room dressing Pictures of people doing the task successfully	Developing self efficacy by showing that others are able to achieve change

TABLE 3 Session outline.

Session	Example training activity	Energy level	BCT	Capability Physical	Capability Psychological	Opportunity Physical	Opportunity Social	Motivation Reflective	Motivation Automatic
Hello and welcome 15 min	Introduce the course and yourself	Low energy	Credible source					▓	
Introduce each other 25 min	Fun activity for people to introduce themselves to each other, e.g. *Participant Bingo*: find someone who likes to eat mangos, has a pet, practices yoga, favourite colour is purple etc.	Mid energy							
Setting ground-rules and ways of working together 10 min	Place a simple set of ground rules on a PowerPoint or graffiti sheet. In small groups discuss some of the key ground-rules, e.g. confidentiality, respect, listening, not interrupting, switching off phones. Ask them to feedback thoughts, changes or additions	Threes, then as a whole group Low energy							
What do people know about the behaviour 20 min	Show two video clips of people washing hands. Ask participants to see if they can spot the mistakes made in hand washing in these clips. This will include the process of hand washing as well as the contexts in which hand washing takes place, e.g. after seeing each patient, after touching equipment	Middle to high energy Competitive Two large groups	Demonstrate behaviour Instruction on how to perform the behaviour	▓	▓				

(Continued)

TABLE 3 (Continued)

Session	Example training Activity	Energy level	BCT	Capability Physical	Capability Psychological	Opportunity Physical	Opportunity Social	Motivation Reflective	Motivation Automatic
What do people know about the consequences of the behaviour 15 min	Provide a set of outcomes and ask participants to match it to statements that are placed around the wall. Then discuss as a group. For example **Outcomes** Decreased by 50% £X per day 20% .... **Statements:** Staff absenteeism reduced by. Loss of earnings reduced by. Reduced infection spread by. Increased efficacy of antibiotics by...	Individually then as a whole group Low energy	Information about health, social or environmental consequences						
Benefits and Disadvantages 10 min	Place two sheets on the wall with the title on one called Pros and on the other Cons. Assign half the group to one side and half the group to the other. After 5 minutes ask them to swap. At the end of the exercise, ask people to talk about the pros and cons and discuss how sometimes the cons may seem to outweigh the pros in terms of the number of cons, but on the whole, the value of the pros often are more important. You can have a conversation about what is most important to the health service to assist this discussion	In two groups Mid energy	Pros and cons						

The behaviour 10 min	Now that people have had a chance to consider consequences and advantages/disadvantages of the behaviour it's worth specifying a very clear goal. Ask them to think of their own contexts and to think of a specific goal for that work context. They can write this on flipcharts on the wall starting each sentence with I will wash my hands....	Whole group Mid energy	Goal setting					
Problem solving 25 min	Hand out several small sheets of paper and ask each person to write down one problem on each sheet of paper. Place all the small sheets of paper into a hat. Now ask one person to take ONE problem out of the hat. Write that problem on the graffiti sheet and then brainstorm solutions to that problem. As a group select the problem that can seem the most likely to work. Work your way through that problem. Who would need to do things differently? Be very precise in describing what the solution looks like. **For example:** Problem: Many of my colleagues think that I use too much gel and it is costing the department. Solution: I will have a discussion with my colleagues showing them the information about health and absentee consequences. I will ask them if they can think of solutions? Note: I would normally start this activity with a session on problem solving.	Individually then in groups Mid energy	Problem solving					

(Continued)

TABLE 3 (Continued)

Session	Example training Activity	Energy level	BCT	Capability Physical	Capability Psychological	Opportunity Physical	Opportunity Social	Motivation Reflective	Motivation Automatic
Prompts and Cues 15 min	Discuss prompts: what sorts of things prompt people – posters, items, people, noises, actions? Now: Ask the participants to set out the room as if it was a ward OR provide a large picture of a ward (find someone in the group who likes drawing?). Ask people to place hand hygiene prompts around the ward	Whole group High energy	Prompts and cues						
Practicing the behaviour and the contexts of the behaviour 40 min	**Tag role play** Ask people to now test out what has been achieved so far including problem solving and prompts and cues. Set up the room to mimic a clinic. One person will be the clinician and three people will be patients and one person will be an obstructive clinician. The clinician starts his or her rounds and demonstrates hand washing. This carries on for 3 minutes, then another person takes the clinicians place. As people swap places discuss how easy it was to implement the changes and how effective the prompts and cues were. Where there was an obstructive clinician, what sorts of things helped to gain support?	Whole group High energy	Behavioural practice and rehearsal						

Just one thing **30 min**	Stories about others' approval. Listen to short stories about people's experiences of infection. What one thing could have been done to minimise the risk of infection? Role play a discussion with that person to demonstrate the changes that are being made on the ward	Individually Low energy followed by whole group mid energy	
Making plans **40 min**	Each person to make an action and coping plan for the behaviour and write a series of implementation intentions. Ask them to look at their original goals in order to do so. Discuss these with a colleague. Finally, ask them How will they know if they have been successful? How they will review? When will they review? Who else will know?	Individually Low energy	
Finish **10 min**	Put all the names of individuals in a hat three times, including yourself. Ask individuals to take names out of the hat and to write a thank you to that person about how their input has helped them to learn during the course, or how they will help to support them after the course	Individual and Whole group reflection Low energy	

Example 2   'Let's talk about mental health' (3-hour session).

AIMS

An online course for staff across primary care, community services, acute care, social care and voluntary services to enhance their knowledge, skills and confidence to have quality conversations about mental health and well-being with everyone they work with.

TIPS AND EXAMPLES: SETTING UP A SESSION

TABLE 4   Session outline.

Session content	Reasons for inclusion
Intended Behavioural Outcomes (IBOs) After attending the session staff and volunteers will: • Recognise and respond to opportunities to sensitively start conversations about mental health and well-being • Use open questions and respond to cues to further explore mental health and well-being • Use validating conversation techniques (using a conversation acronym) to have meaningful, quality conversations about mental health and well-being • Signpost or refer people to relevant supporting services	Including IBOs at the start of the session so that learners and tutors are in agreement about the purposes of the session and what learners should be aiming to do differently after the session
Pre-course material A video and brief handout on why having mental health conversations is important for the health and well-being of our communities	Developing some reflective motivation for having mental health conversations so that learners attend wanting to change their practice
Delivery set up Online course – The course was advertised via local council, NHS and voluntary sector newsletters, participants were emailed joining instructions on signing up, and Microsoft Teams was the delivery platform for the training. Recommended group size: Up to 20	Considered time and cost efficient at a time where pandemic restrictions fluctuate and many are hybrid working

(Continued)

TABLE 4 *(Continued)*

Session content	Reasons for inclusion
Exploring influences on change A series of scoping activities were undertaken, including interviews and focus groups with colleagues in the NHS, council and voluntary sector to identify barriers and facilitators to staff and volunteers performing the key practice of interest: **having quality conversations about mental health and emotional well-being with service users**. Key influences to address were: **Capability** – Perceived lack of knowledge about mental health and skill to have effective, sensitive conversations about mental health **Opportunity** – Perceived lack of time, lack of a private space to talk, sense that service users wouldn't want them to start conversations about mental health **Motivation** – Perception that it wasn't their role to talk about mental health, fear of making the person feel worse or damaging the professional relationship	Understanding influences on change before the course can direct how much time is spent on different activities in a tight course schedule

TABLE 5 Session plan, activities linked to BCTs and COM.

Session	Example training activity	Energy level	BCT	Capability Physical	Capability Psychological	Opportunity Physical	Opportunity Social	Motivation Reflective	Motivation Automatic
Hello 10 min	Introduce self and experience in the topic, welcome everyone Ask people to unmute, introduce their name, role, how they are today (e.g., choosing from humorous pictures on screen) and one thing they are hoping to get from our session today.	Mid energy Whole group	Credible source Goal setting (behaviour and outcomes)						
Ground rules **Aims** 10 min	Ask group 'how can we work effectively together today'? and agree, e.g. confidentiality, joining in but looking after yourself, only sharing what you feel comfortable with, respecting each other's experiences, views and ideas. Share a slide explicitly setting out the IBOs of the training.	Mid energy Whole group	Goal setting (behaviour)						
Where are we at just now? 15 min	Ask the group to post on Padlet: • What worries do you have about raising and talking about mental health with the people you work with now? • What has helped you do this so far? • How have you already helpfully changed the way you are doing things? Tell them this will be useful to come back to.	Mid energy Whole group	Part of problem solving Antecedents of behaviour						

What do you mean, mental health?
20 min
	Offer a short slide presentation, covering:
	
	• The mental health spectrum, normalising mental health
	• A video normalising that anyone can experience struggles with mental health and short conversations can be life-changing, often with no need for the professional to provide a 'fix' – just listen and make people feel validated.
	• Present audit and feedback data from the local area showing that:
	   ○ Local people in the area want and expect us to ask about their mental health
	   ○ That holistic care leads to better health outcomes in the local area.
		Didactic
		Whole group
			Information about health and social consequences of the behaviour
			
			Information about others' approval
			
			Salience of consequences

IBO 1:+2 Recognising and responding **30 min**	Small group activities • What are signs (feelings, thinking, physical, behaviours) that someone might be struggling with mental health? • What are different ways of starting the conversation sensitively? Feedback to larger group. Present agenda setting tools they can use with clients and discuss with the group when is the right time Small groups practice different scenarios in threes, where they start the conversations in different ways.	Small group Large group	Information about antecedents Instructions on how to perform the behaviour Adding objects to the environment Behavioural practice and rehearsal

(Continued)

TABLE 5 (Continued)

Session	Example training Activity	Energy level	BCT	Capability Physical	Capability Psychological	Opportunity Physical	Opportunity Social	Motivation Reflective	Motivation Automatic
IBO 3: Conversation tools 60 min	Get into pairs, discussing the last useful conversation they had with someone about something they worried about. What did that person do, and not do that was helpful? List the skills they think they need that they already have and how they demonstrate these to colleagues on a day-to-day basis.	Pairs Medium energy	Instructions on how to perform behaviour						
	Introduce an acronym for skills for structuring mental health conversations that they will be following. Demonstrate this in action – two group members read a scripted interaction and others clap, 'raise hand' or ring a bell when they see skills in action	Whole group Higher energy	Self as role model Demonstration of behaviour						
	Experiential exercise on listening blocks – in threes, one person talking about hobby or holiday, other briefed to use listening blocks (e.g. being distracted, trying to fix the problem too soon, trying to change the subject to avoid any emotional sensitivities), observer tries to spot the blocks. As a whole group, discuss the causes of listening blocks and how we can overcome these barriers.	Small group Higher energy Whole group Lower energy	Practice and behavioural rehearsal. Feedback on behaviour. Antecedents of behaviour Problem solving						
	Back to threes, practice having most of a conversation, using realistic scenarios (pre-tailored to their work setting) and using the acronym. Observer to spot skills, encourage constructive, specific feedback.	Small group Medium energy	Graded tasks Practice and behavioural rehearsal Feedback on behaviour						

IBO 4: Signposting and support 20 min	Reflect on experiences and ideas for how to close conversations effectively. Brainstorm sources of support and signposting, giving out a prompt card for local services.	Whole group Medium energy	Information about how to perform the behaviour Adding objects to the environment Prompts and cues
Moving forwards 10 min	Problem-solving exercise, mix up barriers shared previously and offer back – how could they solve them and swap one behaviour with another? Ensure common barriers to do with lack of time, not feeling they are in the right role to talk about mental health, worry about making patients feel worse, are problem solved.	Whole group Medium energy	Problem solving
	Each group member notes down an action plan 'pledge' – what they commit to doing to put their learning into practice, when, where, how and when they'll review their plan. Encouraged to add these to the evaluation form, then the team will post them back to them via email when back at work as a reminder in 1 month.	Individual Medium energy	Action planning Commitment Prompts/cues
	Thanking everyone and share reflections on the day and one way they'll take things forward in their real-life setting.	Whole group Medium energy	Action planning

Cards for Change

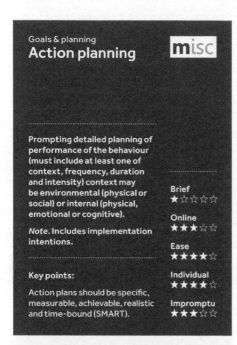

Goals & planning
Action planning

misc

Prompting detailed planning of performance of the behaviour (must include at least one of context, frequency, duration and intensity) context may be environmental (physical or social) or internal (physical, emotional or cognitive).

Note. Includes implementation intentions.

Brief
★ ☆ ☆ ☆ ☆

Online
★ ★ ★ ☆ ☆

Ease
★ ★ ★ ★ ☆

Individual
★ ★ ★ ★ ☆

Impromptu
★ ★ ★ ☆ ☆

Key points:

Action plans should be specific, measurable, achievable, realistic and time-bound (SMART).

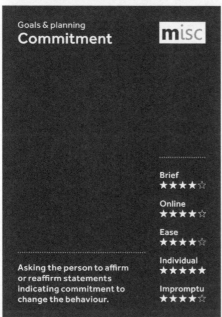

Goals & planning
Commitment

misc

Brief
★ ★ ★ ★ ☆

Online
★ ★ ★ ★ ☆

Ease
★ ★ ★ ★ ☆

Individual
★ ★ ★ ★ ★

Impromptu
★ ★ ★ ★ ☆

Asking the person to affirm or reaffirm statements indicating commitment to change the behaviour.

Goals & planning
Action planning

Activities:

Making a SMART plan: Ask trainees to write down the wanted behaviour. Ask them to then make a detailed plan of how and when they will perform the behaviour. The plan should be SMART: specifying the behaviour; saying how you will know you've done the behaviour; saying when you will do the behaviour and then checking that the behaviour is realistic and achievable in terms of what and how (intensity, duration, context).

Or: Ask trainees to identify cues that automatically help the behaviour happen in that context. For each cue, ask them to make a simple statement, linking the cue and the behaviour: "if [cue] happens then I will do [behaviour]". This is called an 'if-then' plan.

Key points to make the activities work well:

Trainees should come up with their own plans or at least check that suggested plans are SMART. If-then plans are simple. All action plans can be done individually and online or face-to-face.

Goals & planning
Commitment

Activities:

At the end of the session, ask the trainees to each specify one thing that they will commit to do, after the course. Go around the group and ask each of them to state their commitment, starting with: "I will..."

Or: At the end of the session, ask the trainees to each specify one thing that they will commit to change, after the course. Ask each of them to write their commitment on a postcard starting with: "I will..."

Key points to make the activities work well:

Remind the trainees what a behaviour is (something that you will do) and that their commitment should be to do a specified behaviour. You could send the postcards to the trainees after a specified time to help remind them of their commitment.

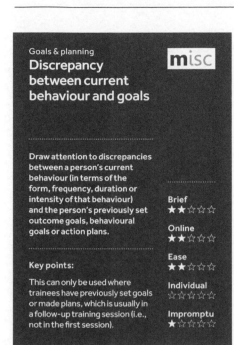

Goals & planning

Discrepancy between current behaviour and goals

Activities:

Ask trainees to discuss to what extent their current behaviour(s) are different to goals (behaviours outcomes or plans). Ask them to estimate a quantifiable discrepancy e.g., a percentage of behaviours that are the same as the goals.

Key points to make the activities work well:

Be cautious about making trainees disclose failures – this should only be done if you are confident that the group feels safe to share information which might provoke negative feelings. You might consider doing this activity one-to-one, or facilitating trainees identifying their own discrepancies without sharing with the group.

Goals & planning

Goal setting (behaviour)

Activities:

Trainer starts the session with the behaviour goal:
Set a behavioural goal at the beginning of a session. For example, you might say 'the goal of this session is to change the way you assess a critically ill patient'.

Trainees set their own individual behaviour goal:
At the end of the session, ask the trainees to think about what changes they are going to make to their practice in line with what they had learned on the course.

Key points to make the activities work well:

Make the goals specific (what will be the behaviour exactly).

Work out how you would know if a behaviour had been done (this is another BCT – monitoring the behaviour).

Behavioural goal setting works well if followed by action planning (another BCT).

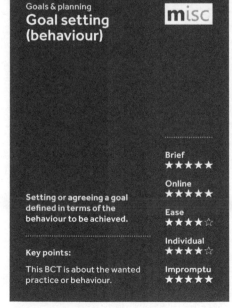

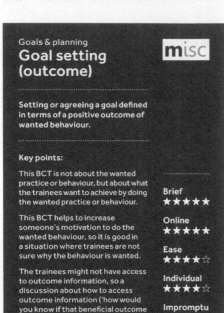

Goals & planning
Goal setting (outcome)

Setting or agreeing a goal defined in terms of a positive outcome of wanted behaviour.

Key points:

This BCT is not about the wanted practice or behaviour, but about what the trainees want to achieve by doing the wanted practice or behaviour.

This BCT helps to increase someone's motivation to do the wanted behaviour, so it is good in a situation where trainees are not sure why the behaviour is wanted.

The trainees might not have access to outcome information, so a discussion about how to access outcome information ('how would you know if that beneficial outcome happened?') might be helpful.

Brief
★★★★★

Online
★★★★★

Ease
★★★★☆

Individual
★★★★☆

Impromptu
★★★★★

Goals & planning
Problem solving

Analysing or prompting the person to analyse, factors influencing the behaviour and generating or selecting strategies that include overcoming barriers and / or increasing facilitators (includes relapse prevention and coping planning).

Key points:

Identifying barriers or facilitators is not enough to be problem solving – solutions also need to be identified.

This BCT helps people who know how to do the behaviour and want to do the behaviour but have either struggled to do it in the past or can foresee lots of difficulties doing it in the future.

Brief
☆☆☆☆☆

Online
★★★☆☆

Ease
★★☆☆☆

Individual
★★★★☆

Impromptu
★★☆☆☆

Goals & planning
Goal setting outcome

Activities:

Trainer starts the session with the outcome goal: Set an outcome goal at the beginning of a session. For example, you might say 'we are here today because you are keen to reduce the number of hospital acquired infections on your ward'.

Trainees set their own individual outcome goal: At the beginning of the course, ask the trainees to think about why they are here and what they want to achieve by changing their practice.

At the end of the course, ask the trainees to think about what would be a good outcome if they made changes to their practice in line with what they had learned on the course.

Key points to make the activities work well:

Make the goals specific (what will be the outcome for whom).

Work out how you could know if a goal had been met.

Goals & planning
Problem solving

Activities:

As small group, simplify and specify problems and solutions: Ask trainees in small groups to identify problems, challenges or to doing the wanted behaviour. Next, ask the group to generate solutions to each of the problems, challenges or barriers. Encourage groups to role-play the solutions e.g., role-play speaking up if you have a concern during an emergency procedure.

The trainees individually work through a list of common barriers and common solutions: Before the training session, create two columns: one of common barriers and one of common solutions to the wanted behaviour(s). Give this to the trainees and ask them to draw a line between barriers and solutions, indicating which solution would help them to overcome each barrier.

Or: Ask each individual to come up with a list of barriers to the wanted behaviour and a list of solutions. Next, ask the trainee to make a list of 'if-then' statements, that link the barriers and solutions.

For example, if the barrier to hand washing was 'no hand wash' and the solution was 'get a bottle of hand wash from store room' the statement would be 'if I get to the sink and the hand wash is not there, then I will go to the store room and get a new bottle'.

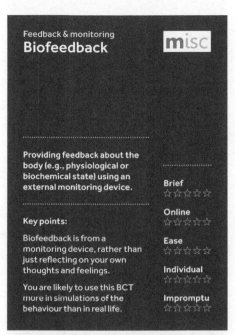

Feedback & monitoring
Biofeedback

misc

Providing feedback about the body (e.g., physiological or biochemical state) using an external monitoring device.

Key points:

Biofeedback is from a monitoring device, rather than just reflecting on your own thoughts and feelings.

You are likely to use this BCT more in simulations of the behaviour than in real life.

Brief
☆☆☆☆☆

Online
☆☆☆☆☆

Ease
☆☆☆☆☆

Individual
☆☆☆☆☆

Impromptu
☆☆☆☆☆

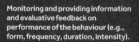

Feedback & monitoring
Feedback on behaviour

misc

Monitoring and providing information and evaluative feedback on performance of the behaviour (e.g., form, frequency, duration, intensity).

Note. If biofeedback, then this is Biofeedback and not this. If feedback is on the outcome of the behaviour, not the behaviour, then this is Feedback on outcome(s) of behaviour and not this.

Key points:

The feedback has to be on the behaviour – so not a generic comment, such as: "that was great".

This BCT is useful when the behaviour is difficult, to help trainees learn and improve the behaviour.

In the workplace, feedback on behaviour might motivate people, by showing approval of the behaviour.

Brief
★★★★★

Online
☆☆☆☆☆

Ease
★★★★★

Individual
★★★☆☆

Impromptu
★★★★★

Feedback & monitoring
Biofeedback

Activities:

Monitoring stress:
If the wanted behaviour is likely to have a positive impact on the stress of the trainee, as seen in a lowering of their heart rate, simulate the scenario for the wanted behaviour, whilst monitoring heart rate with an external heart rate monitor. Simulate the scenario a number of times, sometimes in which the trainee does the wanted behaviour and sometimes in which the trainee does not do the wanted behaviour. Feedback the different heart rates to the trainee.

Key points to make the activities work well:

This activity might work well with activities for reducing negative emotions.

Feedback & monitoring
Feedback on behaviour

Activities:

Using the ALOBA method of feedback:
Just before the trainee is going to practice the behaviour, ask them which specific part of the behaviour they would like feedback on. You could ask a group to offer feedback, too. After the practice, ask the trainee for their own opinion about the behaviour first. Next, offer feedback on the behaviour and ask the group to offer feedback, too.

Key points to make the activities work well:

It is key to create a supportive environment, so that the trainee feels it is OK to reflect on their own areas for improvement.

ALOBA[1] is Agenda-Led Outcome-Based Analysis and it is important that the trainee identifies the feedback they need.

[1]*Silverman JD, Kurtz SM, Draper J.The Calgary-Cambridge approach to communication skills teaching 1: Agenda-led, outcome-based analysis of the consultation. Educ Gen Pract 1996;4:288–299.*

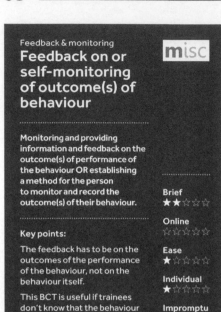

Feedback & monitoring

Feedback on or self-monitoring of outcome(s) of behaviour

Monitoring and providing information and feedback on the outcome(s) of performance of the behaviour OR establishing a method for the person to monitor and record the outcome(s) of their behaviour.

Key points:

The feedback has to be on the outcomes of the performance of the behaviour, not on the behaviour itself.

This BCT is useful if trainees don't know that the behaviour will lead to a desired outcome.

Brief
★★☆☆☆

Online
☆☆☆☆☆

Ease
★☆☆☆☆

Individual
★☆☆☆☆

Impromptu
★☆☆☆☆

Feedback & monitoring

Feedback on or self-monitoring of outcome(s) of behaviour

Activities:

Gathering data on the outcomes of the behaviour: If available to you, gather information on the outcomes of the behaviour (e.g., outcome audit) over time and feed this back to trainees (virtually or face-to-face).

Or: Ask the trainees to think about what evidence is available to them on the desired outcomes from doing the behaviour. Ask them to access or collect that evidence before and after doing the new behaviour; comparing the differences.

Or: When the trainees are simulating / practising the behaviour, offer positive outcome feedback like: "if you did that behaviour in real life then [positive outcome] could have happened".

Key points to make the activities work well:

The outcome of the behaviour can be actual or imagined. Actual outcomes will only be possible where you have contact with the trainees over time or where the activities in the training encourage trainees to get feedback on the outcomes of the behaviour themselves.

Feedback & monitoring

Self-monitoring of behaviour

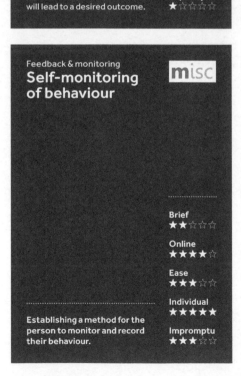

Feedback & monitoring

Self-monitoring of behaviour

Brief
★★☆☆☆

Online
★★★★☆

Ease
★★★☆☆

Individual
★★★★★

Impromptu
★★★☆☆

Establishing a method for the person to monitor and record their behaviour.

Activities:

Providing the trainees with a method for monitoring performance of the behaviour to help them keep track of their behaviour and spot patterns: Give students a reflective log book, in which they record when and where they perform the behaviour.

Or: Organise a brief discussion in which trainees think of ways they could record performance of the behaviour.

Key points to make the activities work well:

Keeping a log of the behaviour might seem like extra work for the trainees. The second activity allows them to think of ways of monitoring which they might find more acceptable.

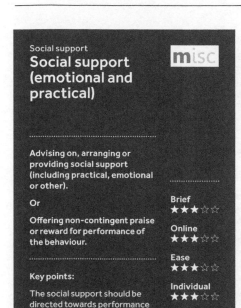

Social support
Social support (emotional and practical)

Activities:

Trainer uses social support with training:
Put the trainees into pairs and ask them to share with each other times when they have done the wanted behaviour(s). Ask them to offer each other general encouragement.

Trainer encourages the use of social support upon return to workplace:
Set up an online forum for people who have attended the course to discuss their experiences of putting the course into practice. You could use 'WhatsApp', 'Facebook' etc.

Key points to make the activities work well:

Activities within sessions should be about generating general, positive support for the new behaviours.

Activities that continue outside the sessions should have ground rules, including expectations of the participants, trainers and others and should be focused on providing positive social support.

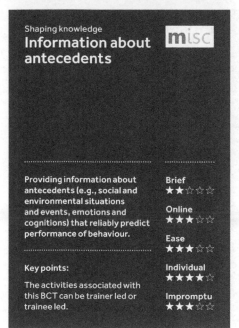

Shaping knowledge
Information about antecedents

Activities:

Including information about antecedents in training:
Prepare materials which detail the kind of events, emotions, and / or conditions that cause or come before the behaviour. For example, you might show evidence that poor team communication (the behaviour) happens when people are tired or when it is noisy.

Asking trainees to keep a record of antecedents:
Where you don't know what reliably precedes the behaviour, ask the trainees to keep a log of when they perform the behaviour and what was happening (thoughts, feelings, surroundings) immediately before the behaviour.

Key points to make the activities work well:

This activity could work well as an activity in an online course, or a face-to-face activity with a group or individually. This BCT links well with self-monitoring of behaviour.

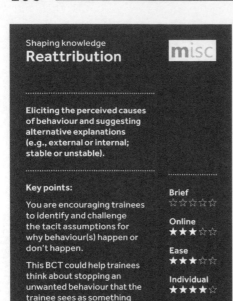

Shaping knowledge
Reattribution

misc

Eliciting the perceived causes of behaviour and suggesting alternative explanations (e.g., external or internal; stable or unstable).

Key points:

You are encouraging trainees to identify and challenge the tacit assumptions for why behaviour(s) happen or don't happen.

This BCT could help trainees think about stopping an unwanted behaviour that the trainee sees as something that is caused by something external to them.

Brief ☆☆☆☆☆

Online ★★★☆☆

Ease ★★★☆☆

Individual ★★★★☆

Impromptu ★★☆☆☆

Shaping knowledge
Reattribution

Activities:

Trainer helps trainees identify assumptions about causes of behaviour: Ask trainees to discuss why the wanted behaviour has not been happening or why the unwanted behaviour has been happening. Next, challenge the group to come up with alternative explanations for the causes.

Including common attributions of the behaviour and challenges in materials: You could include some common attributions with alternative explanations, when you prepare didactic or online materials.

Key points to make the activities work well:

You could make this activity easier by including an example: "often people say behaviours don't change because of time pressures, but what could other explanations be?"

This activity could cause distress as it asks people to identify weaknesses in themselves or others. Ensure there is trust within the group and that there are other activities that focus on the trainees' strengths. Trainers can build trust by not assuming the role of expert in the solutions.

This activity works best when trainees reflect on their own attributions and generate their own alternative explanations (either individually or in a group) or those of others.

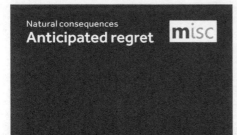

Natural consequences
Anticipated regret

misc

Inducing or raising awareness of expectations of future regret about performance of the unwanted behaviour.

Key points:

This is about imagining the potential future negative consequences of doing the unwanted behaviour or not doing the wanted behaviour.

Brief ★★★☆☆

Online ★★★★☆

Ease ★★★☆☆

Individual ★★★★★

Impromptu ★★★★☆

Natural consequences
Anticipated regret

Activities:

After you have identified an unwanted behaviour, ask trainees to think about how they would feel if they did that behaviour in real life.

Key points to make the activities work well:

This activity could work well as a brief instruction in an online course, or a face-to-face activity with a group.

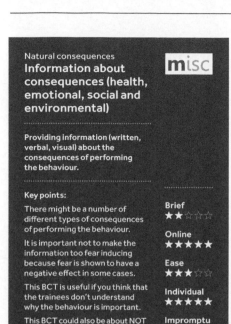

Natural consequences
Information about consequences (health, emotional, social and environmental)

Providing information (written, verbal, visual) about the consequences of performing the behaviour.

Key points:

There might be a number of different types of consequences of performing the behaviour.

It is important not to make the information too fear inducing because fear is shown to have a negative effect in some cases.

This BCT is useful if you think that the trainees don't understand why the behaviour is important.

This BCT could also be about NOT doing a behaviour that is beneficial.

Brief ★★☆☆☆
Online ★★★★★
Ease ★★★☆☆
Individual ★★★★★
Impromptu ★☆☆☆☆

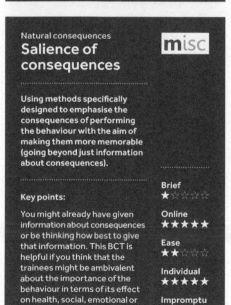

Natural consequences
Salience of consequences

Using methods specifically designed to emphasise the consequences of performing the behaviour with the aim of making them more memorable (going beyond just information about consequences).

Key points:

You might already have given information about consequences or be thinking how best to give that information. This BCT is helpful if you think that the trainees might be ambivalent about the importance of the behaviour in terms of its effect on health, social, emotional or other outcomes.

Brief ★☆☆☆☆
Online ★★★★★
Ease ★★☆☆☆
Individual ★★★★★
Impromptu ☆☆☆☆☆

Natural consequences
Information about consequences (health, emotional, social and environmental)

Activities:

Training includes information in didactic session: In your didactic teaching, include information about how the behaviour(s) are linked to health, emotional, social and / or environmental consequences. You could show some slides, use handouts, use film or photographs.

Key points to make the activities work well:

Prepare material in advance and include both facts and figures, and stories from real people.

Make the information clear and link the consequences clearly to the wanted behaviour(s).

Natural consequences
Salience of consequences

Activities:

Training includes some group reflection on the consequences: Ask your group to talk about any experiences they have where the wanted behaviour (or lack of it) had consequences. This allows people to use their own stories, which are often salient to a group of similar trainees.

Didactic information includes personal experiences, films, photographs: When preparing your information about consequences, try to use materials which bring the information to life. This might be photographs, personal stories or videos.

Key points to make the activities work well:

Prepare material in advance and include both facts and figures, and stories from real people.

Link the consequences clearly to the wanted behaviour(s).

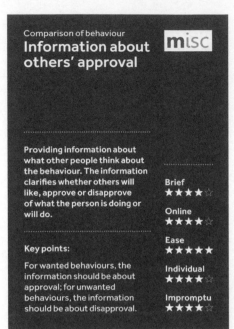

Comparison of behaviour
Information about others' approval

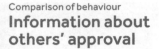

Providing information about what other people think about the behaviour. The information clarifies whether others will like, approve or disapprove of what the person is doing or will do.

Key points:

For wanted behaviours, the information should be about approval; for unwanted behaviours, the information should be about disapproval.

Brief
★★★★☆

Online
★★★★☆

Ease
★★★★★

Individual
★★★★☆

Impromptu
★★★★☆

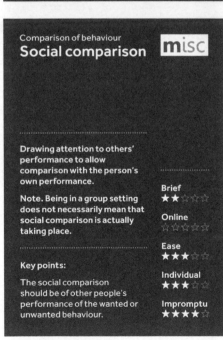

Comparison of behaviour
Social comparison

Drawing attention to others' performance to allow comparison with the person's own performance.

Note. Being in a group setting does not necessarily mean that social comparison is actually taking place.

Key points:

The social comparison should be of other people's performance of the wanted or unwanted behaviour.

Brief
★★☆☆☆

Online
☆☆☆☆☆

Ease
★★★☆☆

Individual
★★★☆☆

Impromptu
★★★★☆

Comparison of behaviour
Information about others' approval

Activities:

Prepare materials which detail how others approve of the wanted behaviour and / or disapprove of the unwanted behaviour. This could be a story in a video, written narratives or evidence from surveys which show how others perceive the behaviour.

Key points to make the activities work well:

We know that information is persuasive if it contains both narrative and facts and figures. Your material could include interviews (video or written) with people about the behaviour and also some facts about others approval or disapproval.

Comparison of behaviour
Social comparison

Activities:

Prepare material which shows rates of performance of the wanted or unwanted behaviour in people similar to the trainees. Share the material with the trainees and ask them to compare their own performance of the behaviour with the others.

Or: Ask the trainees to think about someone they admire and their performance of the behaviour. Ask them to reflect (write down, discuss in a group or in pairs) on their performance of the behaviour compared to the person they admire.

Key points to make the activities work well:

The first activity will work best if there is an opportunity for trainees to bring evidence of their own performance (e.g., audit data) with them and if you have access to relevant data. If these types of data are not available, the second activity will allow some social comparisons without evidence.

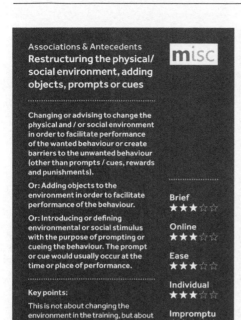

Associations & Antecedents
Restructuring the physical/social environment, adding objects, prompts or cues

Changing or advising to change the physical and / or social environment in order to facilitate performance of the wanted behaviour or create barriers to the unwanted behaviour (other than prompts / cues, rewards and punishments).

Or: Adding objects to the environment in order to facilitate performance of the behaviour.

Or: Introducing or defining environmental or social stimulus with the purpose of prompting or cueing the behaviour. The prompt or cue would usually occur at the time or place of performance.

Key points:

This is not about changing the environment in the training, but about changing things in the workplace.

Brief
★★★☆☆

Online
★★★☆☆

Ease
★★★☆☆

Individual
★★★☆☆

Impromptu
★★☆☆☆

Associations & Antecedents
Restructuring the physical/social environment, adding objects, prompts or cues

Activities:

Mapping the environment and imagining changes for a wanted behaviour:
In a group, ask the trainees to map their physical working environment (you could use drawing, modelling clay, building bricks such as Lego® or other playful learning props). Ask them to model doing the wanted behaviour in the environment and to think about any physical changes that would help them to perform the new behaviour.

Key points to make the activities work well:

Trainees should be encouraged to model the whole environment (physical and social) and to be really creative in thinking about who and what could help in performing the wanted behaviour.

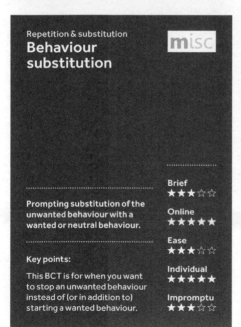

Repetition & substitution
Behaviour substitution

Prompting substitution of the unwanted behaviour with a wanted or neutral behaviour.

Key points:

This BCT is for when you want to stop an unwanted behaviour instead of (or in addition to) starting a wanted behaviour.

Brief
★★★☆☆

Online
★★★★★

Ease
★★★☆☆

Individual
★★★★★

Impromptu
★★★☆☆

Repetition & substitution
Behaviour substitution

Activities:

Ask the trainees to think about what they could do instead of the unwanted behaviour. This could be a new, neutral behaviour or even one of the wanted behaviours in the training. Ask the trainees to think about directly substituting the unwanted behaviour with the new behaviour. They could talk about this: in pairs; groups or think or write about this individually.

Key points to make the activities work well:

This could be done online or face-to-face, in pairs, groups or individually.

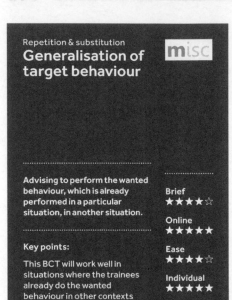

Repetition & substitution

Generalisation of target behaviour

misc

Advising to perform the wanted behaviour, which is already performed in a particular situation, in another situation.

Brief
★★★★☆

Online
★★★★★

Key points:

This BCT will work well in situations where the trainees already do the wanted behaviour in other contexts but you want them to in other situations too.

Ease
★★★★☆

Individual
★★★★★

Impromptu
★★★☆☆

Repetition & substitution

Graded tasks

misc

Setting easy-to-perform tasks, making them increasingly difficult but achievable, until behaviour is performed.

Key points:

This BCT will work only if you have repeated contact with the trainees, in between which they have opportunities to perform the wanted behaviour.

This is different to the gradual development of a skill (which is becoming ABLE to do the skill, rather than actually DOING the skill in real life).

This BCT is suitable for tasks that the trainees think are hard to perform.

Brief
☆☆☆☆☆

Online
★★★☆☆

Ease
★★★☆☆

Individual
★★★★☆

Impromptu
☆☆☆☆☆

Repetition & substitution

Generalisation of target behaviour

Activities:

Identify the wanted behaviour and ask the trainees to think about times when they do the wanted behaviour already. Ask them to think about the contexts or situations in which they do the wanted behaviour. Identify the new situations in which you want them to perform the wanted behaviour.

Key points to make the activities work well:

This activity could be face-to-face, online, in a group or individual.

Repetition & substitution

Graded tasks

Activities:

Ask trainees in a group to think about the wanted behaviour and whether it is manageable for them. For behaviours that the trainees think are difficult or are concerned will not be manageable, ask them to think about a behaviour that is not quite the wanted behaviour but that is manageable.

Key points to make the activities work well:

Only attempt this, if the trainees think the behaviour is difficult but that there are steps that might build up to the behaviour. For example, trainees might find taking an ABCDE approach to illness management hard, but might feel confident in assessing airway and then calling for help. Encourage them to make that first step. The graded tasks rely on ongoing contact with the trainees, so that the tasks can gradually increase in difficulty until target behaviour is achieved.

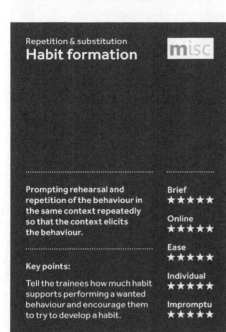

Repetition & substitution
Habit formation

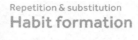
misc

Prompting rehearsal and
repetition of the behaviour in
the same context repeatedly
so that the context elicits
the behaviour.

Key points:

Tell the trainees how much habit
supports performing a wanted
behaviour and encourage them
to try to develop a habit.

Brief
★ ★ ★ ★ ★

Online
★ ★ ★ ★ ★

Ease
★ ★ ★ ★ ★

Individual
★ ★ ★ ★ ★

Impromptu
★ ★ ★ ★ ★

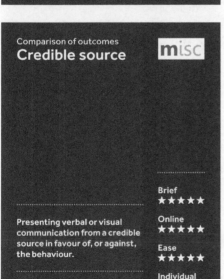

Comparison of outcomes
Credible source

misc

Presenting verbal or visual
communication from a credible
source in favour of, or against,
the behaviour.

Key points:

The point of this BCT is not
what is said, but who is saying it.

Brief
★ ★ ★ ★ ★

Online
★ ★ ★ ★ ★

Ease
★ ★ ★ ★ ★

Individual
★ ★ ★ ★ ☆

Impromptu
★ ★ ★ ★ ★

Repetition & substitution
Habit formation

Activities:

Tell the trainees how much habit can help them
to do the wanted behaviour. Ask them to try to
do the new behaviour over again, many times,
when they return to their work place. Ask trainees
to shout out times when the wanted behaviour
will be appropriate so that they can share ideas
between each other.

Comparison of outcomes
Credible source

Activities:

If you have credible sources within the trainers,
ask them to introduce themselves stating explicitly
why they are experts in the behaviours featured in
the training.

You could prepare materials which feature stories
from a credible source, including videos, written
narratives and podcasts.

Key points to make the activities work well:

Think about what makes a source credible. This
will be linked to what they are saying. If what they
are saying is about the experience of an outcome
of a behaviour, then you might want patients as
credible sources. If it is about overcoming barriers
or facilitators to preforming a behaviour, you might
want someone like the trainees themselves. If
it is about the social desirability of performing
the behaviour, you might want someone whose
opinions are important to the trainees, for example
a senior person.

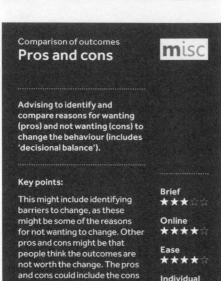

Comparison of outcomes

Comparison of outcomes
Pros and cons

Comparison of outcomes
Pros and cons

Advising to identify and compare reasons for wanting (pros) and not wanting (cons) to change the behaviour (includes 'decisional balance').

Key points:

This might include identifying barriers to change, as these might be some of the reasons for not wanting to change. Other pros and cons might be that people think the outcomes are not worth the change. The pros and cons could include the cons of engaging in change (e.g., the mental resource required to change) as well as those of the new behaviour itself.

Brief
★★★☆☆
Online
★★★★☆
Ease
★★★★☆
Individual
★★★★☆
Impromptu
★★★★☆

Activities:

Ask the trainees to list pros and cons for changing from the current way of doing things to the new way, which would include the wanted behaviour OR exclude the unwanted behaviour.

Key points to make the activities work well:

This activity could be group, individual, face-to-face or online. It might be a really good activity to include to identify barriers and facilitators of changing behaviour and therefore used before planning activities.

Reward & threat
Social reward

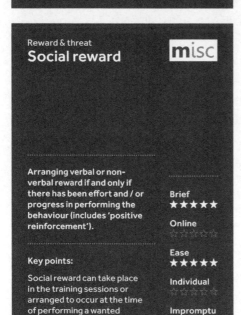

Reward & threat
Social reward

Arranging verbal or non-verbal reward if and only if there has been effort and / or progress in performing the behaviour (includes 'positive reinforcement').

Key points:

Social reward can take place in the training sessions or arranged to occur at the time of performing a wanted behaviour in real life.

Brief
★★★★★
Online
☆☆☆☆☆
Ease
★★★★★
Individual
☆☆☆☆☆
Impromptu
★★★★★

Activities:

Social reward during training:
During the simulation of a scenario in which the wanted behaviour should be used, ask the observing group, and yourself, to notice when the wanted behaviour happens and to congratulate the trainee.

Trainer encourages the use of social reward upon return to work place:
Suggest to trainees that they make efforts to praise other trainees when they observe attempts to perform the wanted behaviour.

Key points to make the activities work well:

The social rewards work best when they are for someone starting to perform a wanted behaviour, so the reinforcement is of the initiation of the behaviour, rather than its successful completion. For example, if a trainee remembered to wash their hands at the correct time, the trainer could say 'it's great that you remembered to wash your hands there'.

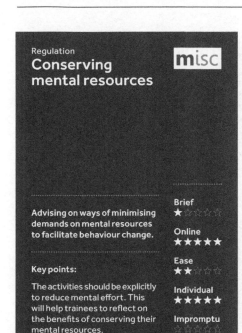

Regulation
Conserving mental resources

misc

Advising on ways of minimising demands on mental resources to facilitate behaviour change.	**Brief** ★☆☆☆☆
	Online ★★★★★
Key points:	**Ease** ★★☆☆☆
The activities should be explicitly to reduce mental effort. This will help trainees to reflect on the benefits of conserving their mental resources.	**Individual** ★★★★★
	Impromptu ☆☆☆☆☆

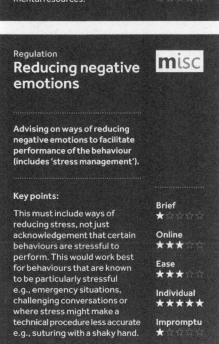

Regulation
Reducing negative emotions

misc

Advising on ways of reducing negative emotions to facilitate performance of the behaviour (includes 'stress management').

Key points:

This must include ways of reducing stress, not just acknowledgement that certain behaviours are stressful to perform. This would work best for behaviours that are known to be particularly stressful e.g., emergency situations, challenging conversations or where stress might make a technical procedure less accurate e.g., suturing with a shaky hand.

Brief ★☆☆☆☆
Online ★★★☆☆
Ease ★★★☆☆
Individual ★★★★★
Impromptu ★☆☆☆☆

Regulation
Conserving mental resources

Activities:

For wanted behaviours where you have identified a high cognitive load as a risk for non-performance:
Highlight a wanted behaviour and ask the group to make a list of all the other things that could be happening when that behaviour should be performed. Reflect back to the group that there are a lot of things going on and that these require mental resource. Ask the group to identify any of the things they've identified that could be done at another time or by another person.

Didactic online information about mental resources:
In your online information, for each wanted behaviour where you have identified a high cognitive load as a risk for non-performance, describe one of these contexts and make suggestions about activities that could be done at a different time or by a different person.

Key points to make the activities work well:

Before any new behaviour becomes routine it can demand effort, and minimising other activities can help. You could use a metaphor e.g., "when you are driving somewhere new, you might turn the radio down to help you concentrate".

Regulation
Reducing negative emotions

Activities:

Practising relaxation whilst simulating the behaviour:
Whilst simulating a behaviour known to elicit negative emotions, ask the person role-playing, and the group, to pause the simulation as a stage at which they think they would feel stress, anxiety or other negative emotions. First, ask the group if any of them have techniques that they use to reduce their negative emotions. If any are volunteered, ask the group to practice them whilst continuing the simulation. If none are volunteered, suggest simple relaxation techniques, such as slowing breathing, focusing on lengthening out breaths or other techniques.

Identifying negative emotions and suggesting techniques:
When preparing information about performing behaviours that are known to elicit negative emotions, identify this as a risk to performing the behaviour and suggest relaxation techniques, like those above.

Key points to make the activities work well:

There are courses, techniques, apps and other resources for reducing negative emotions (including stress management) that you could introduce to your trainees in the activities above.

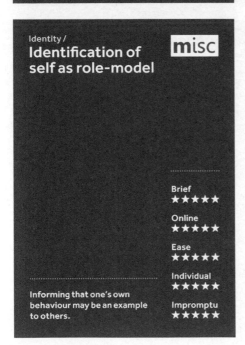

Identity /
Framing/ reframing

misc

Suggesting the deliberate adoption of a perspective on the behaviour (e.g., its purpose) in order to change cognitions or emotions about performing the behaviour (includes 'cognitive structuring').

Key points:

You are helping trainees to think or feel differently about doing the behaviour.

This BCT could help if trainees thought that doing the wanted behaviour was going to be difficult or it might make them feel awkward or uncomfortable.

Brief
★★★★☆

Online
★★★☆☆

Ease
★★★☆☆

Individual
★★★★☆

Impromptu
★★☆☆☆

Identity /
Framing/reframing

Activities:

Trainer helps trainees think in a different way about the behaviour:
Ask trainees to discuss the behaviour and to suggest what they think or feel about doing that behaviour. Next, challenge the group to come up with alternative ways of thinking about the behaviour. For an unwanted behaviour that you want to stop, ask the group whether they had come up with positive thoughts or feelings and whether there were any negative thoughts and feelings associated with the behaviour that they could think of instead. For a wanted behaviour, ask them to do the opposite: identifying any negative feelings and thoughts they've had and asking them to think about any positive thoughts or feelings they could focus on instead.

Including common thoughts or feelings about the behaviour and alternatives in materials:
You could include some common thoughts or feelings (if you know them) with alternative framings alongside them, when you prepare didactic or online materials.

Key points to make the activities work well:
You could model what you expect their thought process to be i.e., "at first I thought.... but now I think...."

Identity /
Identification of self as role-model

misc

Informing that one's own behaviour may be an example to others.

Brief
★★★★★

Online
★★★★★

Ease
★★★★★

Individual
★★★★★

Impromptu
★★★★★

Identity /
Identification of self as role-model

Activities:

Including brief information about the trainee as a role-model:
After trainees have learned about a behaviour, inform them that if they perform the behaviour their colleagues might follow their example. You could identify the group as 'champions'.

An imagination exercise about performing the behaviour:
After trainees have learned about a behaviour, ask them to picture themselves in their workplace doing that behaviour. Ask them to describe what is around them, what is happening and who is there. Next, ask them (or the group) to identify who might be learning from the good practice described.

Key points to make the activities work well:

This first activity could work well as a brief instruction in an online course, or a face-to-face activity with a group.

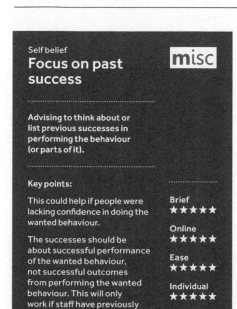

Self belief
Focus on past success

misc

Advising to think about or list previous successes in performing the behaviour (or parts of it).

Key points:

This could help if people were lacking confidence in doing the wanted behaviour.

The successes should be about successful performance of the wanted behaviour, not successful outcomes from performing the wanted behaviour. This will only work if staff have previously tried or known about the wanted behaviour.

Brief
★★★★★

Online
★★★★★

Ease
★★★★★

Individual
★★★★★

Impromptu
★★★★★

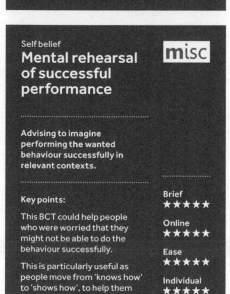

Self belief
Mental rehearsal of successful performance

misc

Advising to imagine performing the wanted behaviour successfully in relevant contexts.

Key points:

This BCT could help people who were worried that they might not be able to do the behaviour successfully.

This is particularly useful as people move from 'knows how' to 'shows how', to help them think about the steps involved in successfully performing the wanted behaviour.

Brief
★★★★★

Online
★★★★★

Ease
★★★★★

Individual
★★★★☆

Impromptu
★★★★★

Self belief
Focus on past success

Activities:

Including brief instructions to focus on past success:
After activities to learn about or rehearse the behaviour, ask staff to shout out or talk in a small group about their previous successes in performing the wanted behaviour.

Key points to make the activities work well:

You could use an example like "the times you managed to disinfect your hands, what might have been the positive results of this? Did it keep your patient well?"

This activity could work well as a brief instruction in an online course, or a face-to-face activity with a group.

Self belief
Mental rehearsal of successful performance

Activities:

Including brief instructions to mentally rehearse the successful performance:
After trainees have learned about how to perform the behaviour, ask them to mentally go through all the steps of actually doing the behaviour successfully, focusing on the positive emotions involved. You can ask them to rehearse how they would do the behaviour in different contexts.

Key points to make the activities work well:

This activity could work well as a brief instruction in an online course, or a face-to-face session, but is an individual mental rehearsal, so is appropriate to do individually.

Sometimes behaviours are easy to do in some contexts and not so in others, possibly because of opportunity barriers. Ask the trainees to rehearse doing the behaviour in all the contexts they will have to do the behaviour.

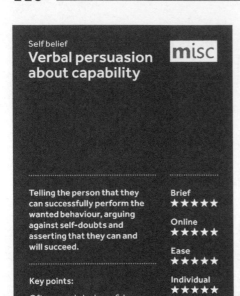

Self belief
Verbal persuasion about capability

misc

Telling the person that they can successfully perform the wanted behaviour, arguing against self-doubts and asserting that they can and will succeed.

Key points:

Often people lack confidence or feel despondent if they find the wanted behaviour difficult.

Brief
★★★★★

Online
★★★★★

Ease
★★★★★

Individual
★★★★★

Impromptu
★★★★★

Self belief
Verbal persuasion about capability

Activities:

Look out for a trainee expressing (verbally or non-verbally) that they are not sure whether they can do the wanted behaviour. In response, state that they can succeed in doing the wanted behaviour, pointing out how likely they are to be able to do the wanted behaviour, reinforcing that they are capable and competent.

Key points to make the activities work well:

This is not a stand-alone activity, but rather a way of giving positive support to trainees. Phrases like "you are really skilled and these are just small tweaks", "we know you can do this" and "you're very likely to succeed" will help.

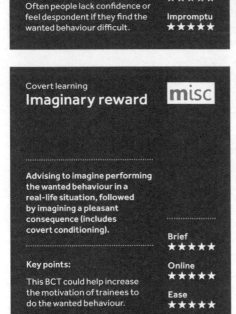

Covert learning
Imaginary reward

misc

Advising to imagine performing the wanted behaviour in a real-life situation, followed by imagining a pleasant consequence (includes covert conditioning).

Key points:

This BCT could help increase the motivation of trainees to do the wanted behaviour.

This is about imagining the positive consequences of doing the behaviour, not about imagining or learning negative consequences.

Brief
★★★★★

Online
★★★★★

Ease
★★★★★

Individual
★★★★★

Impromptu
★★★★★

Covert learning
Imaginary reward

Activities:

Including brief instructions to imagine reward: After trainees have learned about a behaviour, ask them to imagine (themselves) or discuss (in a group) what good things would happen if they did that behaviour in real life. The good things could be for themselves or others.

Key points to make the activities work well: This activity could work well as a brief instruction in an online course, or a face-to-face activity with a group.

Key points to make the activities work well:

You might want to ask trainees to think about what they personally would find rewarding.

Index

Note: Page numbers in *italics* refer to figures; those in **bold** to tables

Training to Change Practice: Behavioural Science to Develop Effective Health Professional Education, First Edition. Jo Hart, Lucie Byrne-Davis, Wendy Maltinsky, and Eleanor Bull.
© 2023 John Wiley & Sons Ltd. Published 2023 by John Wiley & Sons Ltd.